AYURVEDA

AND

PANCHAKARMA

The Science of Healing and Rejuvenation

Sunil V. Joshi, M.D. (Ayu)

LOTUS

DISCLAIMER

This book is not intended to treat, diagnose or prescribe. The information contained herein is in no way to be considered as a substitute for a consultation with a duly licensed health care professional.

Cover art and design: Paul Bond, Art & Soul Design
Illustrations: Margo Gal
Photography: David Hoptman
Design & Page Layout: Carola Höchst-Teague
Editor: Jonathan Crews

First Edition, 1997

Printed in the United States of America

Library of Congress Cataloging-in-Publication-Data
Joshi, Sunil V., 1960
Ayurveda and Panchakarma: The Science of Healing and Rejuvenation/by Dr. Sunil V. Joshi
includes bibliographical references.
ISBN 0-914955-37-3   96-79621
                                                          CIP

Published by:
Lotus Press, P.O. Box 325, Twin Lakes, Wisconsin 53181

DEDICATION

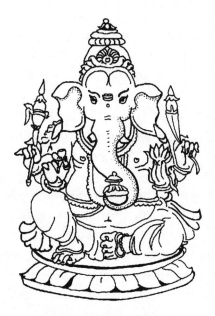

Lord Ganesha

To my loving parents, Vinayak and Shobhana Joshi. You are my great inspiration. Your genuine love and support have encouraged me in this wonderful dharma.

To my wife, Shalmali, and my daughter, Siddha. Your love and support manifest in so many ways, but in particular through your patience and understanding.

Finally, I wish to express my deep gratitude to Dhanvantari, and to the great seers, Charaka and Sushruta, for gifting Ayurveda to the world, and to Shri Ramakrishna and Mataji, my beloved Gurus.

ACKNOWLEDGEMENTS

First and foremost, I wish to express my gratitude to Maharishi Mahesh Yogi, who is responsible for re-enlivening the full potential of Ayurveda and making it available on a worldwide level.

I wish to thank my teachers, Vaidya B. S. Katti, Vaidya B.V. Sathye and Pundit Shivakaran Sharma Chhanganiji, for the knowledge and inspiration which they gave so generously. It was under their tutelage that so many insights into this great science were revealed to me. I am ultimately grateful to the inner guidance that directed me to this fortunate dharma. As a physician, Ayurveda's holistic understanding of health has given me immense satisfaction and an infinitely deep respect for life. After many years of daily clinical practice, I have never wavered in my devotion to it.

I offer my gratitude to Vaidya Bindumadhav Sridhar Katti for motivationg me to practice Ayurveda.

I want to express my sincere thanks to Vaidya B.V. Sathye for giving me insights through his lectures.

I want to express my personal thanks to Lenny Blank and Ivy Blank for introducing me to the West and motivating me to write *Ayurveda and Panchakarma*, also to Lenny Blank for producing this book for Lotus Press.

Sincere thanks to Gerhardt Horstman and Dean Campbell for helping me to expand Panchakarma in the United States and for supporting my success in the West.

A thank you to the following who worked on the production of this book: David Hoptman – Photography; Leslie and James Vogel – Models; Paul Bond – Cover; Margo Gal – Illustrations; John Wozencraft – Charts; Carola Höchst-Teague – Page Layout; and Parvati Markus – Editing.

Below is a list of individuals to whom I would like to express my deep love and warmest regards for their unselfish support:

Deepak Chopra, M.D. (for his valuable contribution in supporting the recognition of Ayurveda by the scientific community and popularizing it throughout the West); Dr. David Frawley (Vamadeva Shastri); David Simon, M.D.; Patrick Hanaway, M.D.; Gabriel Cousens, M.D. (for his support in doing research on Panchakarma therapy); Huntley Dent; Gerri Shafer Smith; Drs. Natarajan A. & Uma N. Iyer; Dr. Vinaykumar S. Golvardhan; Dr. Madhukar S. Pathak; my brothers Mukul and Anil, his wife Anuja and son Abhir, my sister Anjali and her husband Rajendra and children Gaurang and Gayatri Dive, Pravin, my clinic staff in India; all my clients, organizers, and the many others who have made a lasting impression on my life.

Finally, I wish to express my special gratitude to Jonathan Crews for his skillful assistance and guidance in writing this book. Without his total commitment and dedication, this book would not be available to the reader today.

TABLE OF CONTENTS

SECTION I

THE FOUNDATIONS OF AYURVEDA

SECTION II
AYURVEDIC TREATMENT OF DISEASE

Foreword

Human beings are suffering despite access to technological advances that offer the promise of unequaled improvements in our quality of life. The flaws in our reliance on a materially-based approach to health are increasingly apparent. Despite amazing diagnostic machines and designer-crafted medicines, our society is suffering from preventable epidemics of heart disease, cancer and infectious illnesses. Of equal importance is the recognition that a large segment of our population, while not demonstrating full-blown evidence of disease, is nevertheless not living a true state of health.

In this context, Ayurveda, the ancient system of healing from India, has captured the attention and imagination of the West. The message of Ayurveda is simple: health is more than the mere absence of a definable disease; rather, it is the dynamic integration between our environment, body, mind and Spirit. Health is the return of wholeness and ultimately reflects a higher state of consciousness. Within this framework, all healing systems can find a home.

Ayurveda teaches that we are not passive victims of pathogenic forces, but can substantially impact our quality of life through the choices and interpretations we make. By reducing the toxins and increasing the nourishing influences we ingest, we can transform our minds and bodies.

As the science of life, Ayurveda is an inexhaustible reservoir of information. Throughout the ages, devoted explorers of this ocean of wisdom have integrated their personal experiences and interpretations with Ayurvedic knowledge to create something which is simultaneously timeless and modern. Dr. Sunil Joshi has continued this venerable tradition with his book, *Ayurveda and Panchakarma*.

For the past several years, Sunil Joshi has been my teacher, spiritual brother and friend. As one of the foremost experts on Panchakarma, Dr. Joshi has vast experience with the clinical application of this profound science of purification. As a willing and gifted teacher, Dr. Joshi offers pearls of wisdom that can be treasured by both beginners and advanced practitioners. The sharing of his insights on Panchakarma is unprecedented in the English language and provides a firm foundation for understanding and implementing this valuable aspect of Ayurveda. I view this book as a sweet gift of love from Dr. Joshi to the world and I am sincerely grateful to him for his humble contribution to healing the world.

David Simon, M.D.
Medical Director
The Chopra Center for Well Being

INTRODUCTION

I come from India, land of the *Veda*. For longer than mankind can remember, India has been the custodian of this timeless wisdom of the totality of life. From the perspective of *Vedic* knowledge, no aspect of life is disconnected from its source. Every expression of human endeavor, whether it be music, art, architecture, mathematics, agriculture or medicine, is structured in the eternal laws of nature which govern and order our existence.

As a child growing up in India, I had a traditional education and was exposed to many aspects of these *Vedic* sciences, but the area that really captured my imagination was health. From a young age I was fascinated by the human body. I wanted to see inside it and find out how it worked. I would often sneak into hospitals and, from hidden vantage points, watch the doctors perform surgery. I also realized, even as a boy, that I had a strong desire to ease the suffering of others.

Seeing my preoccupation with health, my father told me the story of my great, great grandfather, Shankarji Joshi. Shankarji was a famous *vaidya*, or Ayurvedic physician, renowned throughout India for his skill in this ancient healing science. His entire life was dedicated to bringing health to the people of his area, and he did so until he passed on at the age of ninety-six. It was said that by the time he was sixty-eight, he had lost many of his teeth and his vision had weakened. He went away for a period and underwent *kaya kalpa*, an ancient rejuvenation procedure documented by the Ayurvedic texts, which not only restored his vitality and eye sight, but also gave him back his teeth.

My father once said that at the time of Shankarji's death, he told his son – my father's father– that he would return to bring the knowledge of Ayurveda to his people, and that he would come back as the son of Vinayak, the name given to my dear father. Whether I am, in fact, that great soul, Shankarji, is of little consequence. It is, however, his inspiration burning inside me that guided me to the medical profession.

I did not immediately gravitate toward my great grandfather's calling as a *vaidya*. I entered a school that offered training in both Western (allopathic) and Ayurvedic medicine and had to decide between them. Both my parents worked hard as educators, but were not well paid for their efforts. As the eldest son, I wanted to make their life comfortable and financially secure. Western medicine promised greater financial security, adding this incentive to my long fascination with surgery

Around the time that I received my medical degree in Ayurveda my mother became acutely ill. For years she had suffered from amoebiasis, a parasitic infection common throughout India. Treatment by allopathic doctors had only temporarily alleviated her symptoms. Finally, the amoebas had invaded her liver and formed cysts, causing her to enter a life-threatening phase of the disease called amoebic hepatitis. She was admitted to the hospital for intensive care. However, as a result of being treated with powerful but toxic drugs, she began to experience a range of new symptoms, including further metabolic breakdown, leg pain, and headaches. She was so depressed that she begged us to remove her from the hospital. Feeling confused and in fear for her life, we brought her home.

A family friend suggested that we take her to a local Ayurvedic practitioner. We saw this as a last resort, but we had nowhere else to turn. After a thorough examination, Dr. Katti, the Ayurvedic physician, gave her some herbal preparations and strict dietary guidelines. In three weeks she had completely recovered. Now, many years later, my mother maintains good health and still takes care of her family.

I was deeply affected when I saw my mother respond so quickly to such a simple treatment program after years of suffering through unsuccessful allopathic therapies. My father reminded me that this ancient system of health-care was my heritage, handed down to me from my great, great grandfather. I began to reconsider my direction in medicine. Now that I had my M.D. in Ayurveda, I had to select an area of medicine for postgraduate study and specialization. Until this point, I was committed to pursuing modern medicine, but I started having second thoughts about Western medicine. I was aware of its many achievements, but was also painfully familiar with its shortcomings, especially the deleterious side effects of many of its therapies and the high cost to patients and their families. An inner voice encouraging me to investigate Ayurveda grew stronger in my heart and I decided to study it in depth at the All India Research Institute in Nagpur, a city in central India.

I already knew about some of the significant differences between Ayurveda and the Western approach to diagnosis and treatment. However, as I probed more deeply into Ayurvedic theory and clinical practice, I became impressed by its logic and charmed by the power and completeness of its comprehensive understanding of life. It described a vital connection between individual life and the whole of nature; human life was perceived as a microcosm or intimate reflection of the entire universe.

As I continued my studies, I became fascinated by the area of Ayurvedic science known as *Panchakarma*, a comprehensive system of knowledge and practices to purify the body of toxins and restore it to balance with natural law. In case after case, I watched *Panchakarma* achieve complete remission of disease in patients who could not be helped by Western medicine. In addition, I saw how this science of purification and rejuvenation could take a person with relatively normal health and produce a dramatically greater state of health, happiness and fulfillment. In fact, Ayurveda aims to establish the ability to live every aspect of life to its fullest, in complete conscious connection to nature's infinite intelligence, a state often referred to as enlightenment.

When I first arrived in America, I wondered how different the health concerns would be from those of my country. Aside from the higher incidence of drug and alcohol addiction, psychological imbalance and emotional abuse that seemed to be typical of the West, the problems I began to see were remarkably similar. It seems that no country has been able to escape the negative impact of technological life. The increasingly fast pace of modern life, the growing environmental degradation and the loss of connection to the natural rhythms of life are taking their toll on health and happiness everywhere.

As more and more people are falling prey to the adverse effects of stress, I hear more frequent complaints of disturbed sleep, chronic indigestion, poor elimination and lower back pain. Lack of physical and sexual vitality, chronic fatigue, allergies and the inability to either lose or gain weight are also very common problems. Perhaps the most serious side effect of this growing health crisis in the world is the unhappiness that I witness on the faces of the people who come to see me. So many express strong dissatisfaction with their jobs or relationships and seem to have lost their motivation and enthusiasm for life. As a consequence, anxiety and depression have become all too common.

Almost everyone I see has expressed some feeling of frustration with the health-care systems that are available, invariably remarking that they have tried everything and nothing seems to work. One system might address their complaint as a structural misalignment, another as a biochemical imbalance, and still another as a blockage in the flow of energy. One program recommends fasting, stringent dieting or exercise routines, while others prescribe potent vitamin, mineral or medication therapies.

Though each of these approaches has a convincing logic and may be temporarily successful in alleviating the problem, the symptoms eventually reappear. When this happens, the disappointed patient will then move on to the next health practitioner seeking relief. However, the goal of health and wellness will never be realized if they do not address the root cause of their illness.

The limitations of these health-care practices are not necessarily the fault of the particular system nor the people who practice them. Rather the deficiency lies in the basic slant on health that has been imparted by the objective, scientific orientation that fostered them. In this view of life, matter is given primacy and reality is determined on the basis of sensory experience. In other words, if it can be seen with the naked eye or with the aid of a microscope in a laboratory setting, it is deemed to be real or have validity. Even though this "material" world view has emerged relatively recently in our history, its compelling logic and technological significance has catapulted it into a position of dominance in the world.

When we apply this "objective" logic to the understanding of ourselves and our health, however, at least two significant limitations become apparent. First, it creates an artificial distinction between the observer and the observed. In the real world, nothing exists in isolation and therefore cannot be studied out of context with the rest of life. We cannot separate our body and its functioning from the bigger whole, i.e., the other parts of ourselves as well as the world around us.

Secondly, and very closely related, is the fact that much of life as we experience it is non-material. There is nothing tangible about the things we call the mind, the soul and the spirit, even the senses. Yet these things exert a very noticeable influence on the course of our physical existence. A great many general practitioners acknowledge that the majority of the illnesses they treat in their daily practices have psycho-somatic origins. This means that most diseases are caused or complicated by problems which arise in the mind, an aspect of human life that has no real "objective" reality.

Though many people are beginning to sense the limitation of a strictly body-based approach to their health, they are confused about which way to turn. How do you make your way through the maze of fragmented approaches to find a system that truly works to bring you health, vitality and happiness?

I invite you now to entertain a new, and yet very ancient, view of life and health. In this process, you will not be asked to discard your objective orientation but to expand upon it. This is an intuitive, holistic model of health, where the intangible, as well as the more material aspects of life, are given equal importance, for both are considered to be fundamental to life's wholeness.

Ayurveda is a science that is widely acknowledged to be the world's oldest system of health. It is an oral tradition that has been passed down from generation to generation. Only in the last 5000 years was it actually written down. The word Ayurveda comes from the Sanskrit roots *ayu* and *veda*, or, "life" and "knowledge." Thus in the name "Ayurveda," we find its essential meaning and purpose – the complete knowledge of how to live daily life in harmony with cosmic life.

Ayurveda is not just a health-care system but a complete approach to living. It offers a rich and comprehensive conception of life and health that takes into account all parts of human existence, from its most abstract, transcendental value to its most concrete expressions in human physiology. In addition, it clearly upholds the intimate connection between human life and cosmic life.

Why has this ancient paradigm withstood the test of time and continued to this day to be a successful approach to health-care? The first and foremost reason is that it is based on principles which are as old as life itself and are intimately tied to how nature functions everywhere in creation. There are at least seven basic concepts that help to define Ayurveda as a unique and complete "science of life." Some of these may seem initially to be a bit foreign, as they are not a part of modern, scientific thought. But as they are elaborated upon in the succeeding chapters, you will come to appreciate the profound and comprehensive logic upon which they are based.

1. The Unchanging Nature of Ayurvedic Science

Through the thousands of years that Ayurveda has been in recorded existence, its basic principles have never changed because they derive from universal laws of nature which are eternally true. This contrasts with the modern scientific paradigm, where new theories often render previous understandings completely obsolete within a short period of time.

2. The Subjective Methods of Understanding

One of the most defining features of the Ayurvedic system concerns its methods for deriving knowledge. Ayurveda recognizes that much of life is non-physical and cannot be studied objectively. It therefore incorporates a more subjective or intuitive approach to gaining knowledge in addition to objective means. The unseen intelligence which, for instance, orchestrates the process of growth and differentiation in a fetus or in the healing of a disease cannot be analyzed or investigated by the senses, even with the aid of technological means.

Ayurveda therefore relies on in-depth observation of nature's functioning to understand how the non-physical and the physical aspects of life function in a coordinated fashion. It also recognizes there to be an extremely intimate connection between the processes occurring in nature and those going on inside our bodies. The Ayurvedic practitioner is therefore able to draw comparisons between his observations of life as it functions around him and what is happening with his patient.

This process can be illustrated by the phenomenon of fire. In the physical world, fire can be observed transforming the structure of a substance like wood into something different (ash). The Ayurvedic scientist takes note of this and compares how this same principle in nature works within the body to convert raw food stuffs into nutrients through the aid of digestive enzymes and stomach acids.

3. The Five Element Theory

The third concept which sets Ayurveda apart from other healing modalities is the recognition that human life is part and parcel of nature. The specific intelligences that are responsible for orchestrating the natural world also guide all physiological processes within us.

Ayurveda calls these fundamental principles which guide nature's functioning in creation *mahabhutas* or cosmic elements. They are the underlying intelligences that give rise to the five elements commonly known as space, air, fire, water and earth. These elements are the basic building blocks of nature which are responsible for all physical existence. The coordinated interaction of these elements controls all the functions in creation.

4. The Theory of the Three *Doshas*

One of the most powerful conceptual tools in Ayurveda is the three *dosha* theory. This theory explains how the five elements which make up physical creation dynamically combine to control all processes within the human physiology. These three functional capacities are called: *vata*, the principle governing all motion or movement; *pitta*, which controls all transforming processes; and *kapha*, which is responsible for cohesion, growth and liquefaction. Without any one of these processes, there would be no human life.

5. *Prakruti:* Constitutional Type

The fifth premise of Ayurveda, called *prakruti*, is the most useful tool that this science has to offer for maintaining an ideal state of health. It recognizes that each human being is born with a unique combination of the three *doshas*, and that this natural balance is what is responsible for the physical, mental and emotional differences among people. By identifying and maintaining an individual's *prakruti*, Ayurveda can help each person create his or her own state of ideal health.

6. The Effects of the Seasons

The next major foundation stone of Ayurveda recognizes the very intimate relationship between the individual and all aspects of his or her environment. Ayurveda considers seasonal changes and climatic conditions to have a particularly important effect on health. Each change of season brings shifts in wind conditions, temperature and humidity or rainfall. As the predominance of the elements in the environment change, it will impact the balance of the *doshas* within our bodies. If we can recognize and respond to these environmental changes, we will better be able to maintain a functional homeostasis, an ideal equilibrium of the *doshas* within our bodies.

An example of this might be the greater predominance of the "fire" element that occurs during the summer months. As heat grows in the environment, *pitta dosha* will tend to increase within the body. When this particular functional capacity becomes too predominant, its relationship with the other two *doshas* becomes imbalanced, disrupting various physiological processes. This then causes us to feel acidic, hot, physically uncomfortable and sometimes emotionally irritable. When we possess the knowledge of our *prakruti* or unique body type, these potential imbalances can be easily avoided by making the appropriate changes in our diet and lifestyle.

7. *Panchakarma:* The Science of Rejuvenation

The miracle of the human body is that it has a natural healing intelligence which is capable of constantly rejuvenating itself. However, when *doshic* imbalance and weakened digestive capacity allow toxic impurities to form, this natural capacity of the body gets blocked. To remedy this situation, Ayurveda offers the gift of *Panchakarma*, the "science of rejuvenation." In this process, the body is purified of the degenerating influence of these foreign substances, thus freeing it to naturally exercise its inherent rejuvenative abilities.

Many more key concepts could be listed here, but these seven are sufficient to demonstrate the uniqueness of the Ayurvedic approach. This ancient science has always understood health to be a coordinated functioning of spirit, mind and body in intimate relationship with everything else in creation, material and non-material. It recognizes that human life cannot be separated from cosmic life.

This book has been designed in two sections to reflect the way the original text of Ayurveda, the *Charaka Samhita*, first presented this knowledge. The first section, entitled "The Foundations of Ayurveda," explores in detail the principles which define Ayurveda as a science of life and health. It begins with the Ayurvedic understanding of human life, and proceeds systematically with an elaboration of the five element theory, the three *dosha* theory, and the Ayurvedic understanding of digestion and its important relationship to health. The concept of *prakruti* or unique constitutional type, along with the understanding of *prakruti*-specific diet and lifestyle, are then described to give practical utility to the concept of the three *doshas*. Section I ends with the Ayurvedic understanding of the dietary and lifestyle practices which can help each of us maintain an ideal state of health.

Once the theoretical foundation has been laid, Section II delves more deeply into the Ayurvedic understanding of disease and how to treat it. Entitled "The Ayurvedic Treatment Of Disease," this section begins with an elaboration of the six stages of disease formation and then systematically unfolds the knowledge of *Panchakarma*, the science of rejuvenation. In addition to the theory of how *Panchakarma* works to eliminate the cause of disease, this section offers the interested reader a more detailed understanding of how the three phases of this cleansing and rejuvenative therapy are administered. The book ends with a chapter on procedures we can do at home to bring balance back to our life when we do fall ill.

Ayurveda is the world's oldest existing health-care system. India continued to be the custodian of this complete science of life, even when it was essentially lost to the rest of the world for many centuries, but Ayurveda does not belong only to India. It is a science of health based on universal principles and profound insights into the connection between mind and body and the laws of nature which structure all progress in life. Ayurveda offers health and fulfillment for every man and woman in every culture on earth. It is promising to see that this ancient Vedic wisdom is now becoming more widely available and I feel fortunate to be a part of this revival.

I feel honored and privileged to offer the insights I have gained into the Ayurvedic understanding of life and health, and, in particular, to present the knowledge of *Panchakarma*. I have attempted in all cases to be true to the ancient Ayurvedic texts in my description of this science of purification and rejuvenation. May it inspire you to take the journey to perfect health!

The Foundations of Ayurveda

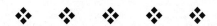

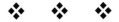

Chapter One

AYU: THE FOUR ASPECTS OF LIFE

W hen discussing the issue of health, it is common for people in all cultures to talk just about their body, its ailments and the medicines they might take to treat these ailments. However, health is not merely a matter of the state of the body, since it is obvious we are much more than just this material form. A system of health that only takes into account the structure and functioning of the physical body cannot effectively address human health in its totality.

Ayurveda is not just a medicinal approach to health. Rather, it is a complete philosophy of life. It gives equal importance to the parts of life which are more subjective and intangible, as well as those which are objective and material, those aspects we can observe with our physical senses. In fact, it is a view of life which understands that the non-material components of our lives — our consciousness, mind, thoughts and emotions — animate and direct our more physical parts.

Based on this perspective, Ayurveda defines *ayu,* or life, as the intelligent coordination of the four parts of life: *atma* (the soul), *manas* (the mind), *indriyas* (the senses) and *sharira* (the body), with the totality of life. Each of these four aspects has specific functions which contribute to the wholeness we experience as life, and Ayurveda focuses on maintaining a balanced, integrated relationship among them. Imbalance, whether physical, mental or emotional, arises when there is a disconnection between the subjective/non-physical and the objective/physical areas of life.

To elaborate on the subjective aspects of human life which

cannot be apprehended by the senses, Ayurveda relies on the tools of observation and comparison, deducing, from the way the universe works, the principles of how the human body functions. Now let's examine each of these four components of life.

ATMA: THE SOUL

The texts of Ayurveda state that in order to fully understand how the body functions, we must first understand the senses and their role in protecting and nourishing the body. Knowledge of the senses, in turn, is gained by understanding the nature of the mind and how it acts to control sensory perception. However, we cannot begin to comprehend the complexity of the human mind unless we understand *atma*, the motivating intelligence that guides the mind as well as all of life. But how did the first Ayurvedic scientists come to understand the nature of this unseen "director" within human life?

Though *atma* is the least tangible part of life, the ancients could identify its existence by the way people always ascribe ownership to things. When people talk, regardless of their cultural background, they refer to aspects of their lives in the possessive case: "My mind is a jumble today"; "My vision is clear"; or "My body feels tired." This implies an inherent duality. There is some aspect within ourselves that possesses a distinct sense of I-ness and sees itself as different from its objects of perception — the mind, the senses and the body — and in ownership of them. These universally common statements reflect *atma* — the sense of "I" as the experiencer — rather than the object of experience, and show that the mind, senses and body are the vehicles through which *atma* gains experience of the world.

The ancients could see that this *atma* or sense of I directed all aspects of human life, but what was the source of this unseen guiding force within each human being? Simple powers of observation were enough to lead them to conclude there was an unimaginable intelligence responsible for creating and orchestrating the vast diversity of the universe. All the various aspects of creation appeared to move together in an intricate interdependency, a wondrous synchrony. It was as if every aspect of life inherently knew how to act in coordination with every other part for the greater good of the whole. This, they deduced, could only occur if every part was, in fact, infused with or connected to that intelligence which had knowledge of the whole.

Through extensive observation of nature and comparison to human life they deduced that this same governing principle existed as a part of us, guiding all mental, sensory and physical processes. As in nature, this intangible director within also had two aspects. The first they identified as *jiva atma* — the quality of innate intelligence usually associated with the concept of "soul" or individual consciousness within us. It imparts the sense of I-ness or individual identity. It can be thought of as our finely tuned guidance system which steers us through life according to our particular destiny.

These early Ayurvedic scientists realized that *jiva atma* or individual soul could have no real existence except in relation to that which gave rise to it. They called this universal quality of intelligence within us *param atma* or "universal soul" and understood it to be the very consciousness of nature. *Param atma* is the very essence of our individual soul, as well as that of everything in creation, and is responsible for animating and unifying all diversity.

The sages compared the relationship that existed between individual soul and universal soul to be like that of the ocean and its waves. *Jiva atma* is an expression of *param atma* in the same way that the wave is an expression of the ocean. Moreover, just as the ocean does not cease to be the ocean when it rises up into a wave, consciousness does not lose its universal status when it individuates into unique expressions of human intelligence. Every *jiva atma* or individual soul, no matter how different it appears to be from every other *jiva atma*, is, in its essential nature, one and the same as the infinite organizing power of *param atma*.

As a unique expression of universal intelligence, each *jiva atma* displays a distinct set of preferences and predispositions. These inherent tendencies serve to guide the soul to achieve its life's purpose. Based on the evolutionary nature of life, the ancients recognized that the ultimate purpose of each soul is to consciously reconnect with that which is its source.

Dharma is the term Ayurveda uses to describe the idea of the soul's special purpose and path. Each soul's inherent preferences lead it to make choices which are consistent with its *dharma*. The soul's powerful will to reconnect the parts of life with the whole of life is what moves human life in an evolutionary, progressive direction. A life that is lived in accord with *dharma* is a life that is in harmony with *ayu*, the totality of life.

The most obvious sign that life is being lived in accord with *dharma* is the joy that comes from doing those things that are most closely aligned with our soul's purpose. Because increasing joy informs us of our proximity to our *dharma* or life's purpose, the soul is ever discriminating among experiences — choosing those experiences that give more happiness, knowledge and satisfaction, and avoiding those that give pain and a feeling of lack.

The ancients found other evidence for the presence of this non-dimensional director of life in identical twins. Two bodies are formed in the same womb, at the same time, with the same genetic material and the same environmental influences, and are born only a few minutes apart. Yet these two individuals will show dramatically different preferences and predispositions in their lives. With all the physical influences being identical, only the presence of souls with distinct predilections could account for these differences.

They also saw evidence of *jiva atma* in the food choices made by an expectant mother. A woman has her own lifelong preferences for certain foods. Yet, when she becomes pregnant, she often begins to desire entirely new things. She may also begin to dislike the foods which she has always enjoyed. What accounts for these changes? It is the new soul in her womb with its own set of desires and preferences which begins to influence the mother's food choices. After the birth of the child, the mother is seen to revert to her normal preferences.

The changes in preferences immediately preceding death further demonstrated to these early physicians the existence of the *jiva atma*. Within twenty-four to forty-eight hours of death, an individual will lose all his or her usual predilections, likes and dislikes. According to the Ayurvedic understanding of the dying process, the soul at this time begins to withdraw from the body, thus explaining the loss of preferences usually associated with that particular soul.

MANAS: THE MIND

If the preferences of the soul are always guiding us on the path to perfect health and wholeness, why do we often make choices which are not conducive to our physical health or our mental and emotional well-being? Why, for example, are we sometimes able to easily control our intake of sugar while at other times we are not, even though we know that too many sweets are not good for us and can cause health problems like obesity, allergies or diabetes? And why, at still other times, do we become completely oblivious to the ramifications of eating sweets and consume them wildly and unconsciously?

This same question can be used to illustrate basic differences between people. Why is it that some people inherently know what is good for them and always act accordingly while others give in to their cravings or addictions in spite of having this knowledge? And why are there still others who do not seem to have a clue about what is best for them?

Ayurveda asserts that all health or ill-health, happiness or unhappiness, and use of our creative potential or not, arises first in the mind. Even though the soul is the director of life, quietly guiding it towards its ultimate destiny, the mind is the controller of the senses and body and determines whether they are used for life's upliftment or degradation. It is the mind that is ultimately responsible for maintaining the harmony between the parts of human life and the universal intelligence that orchestrates all of life. This is why Ayurveda gives *manas* or mind such central importance.

When we lose consciousness of our connection to *atma*, our lives are like that of a storybook prince who develops amnesia and wanders away into the forest, far away from his palace. His survival becomes dependent on the meager roots and berries he can find to feed himself and a small hut of bark he constructs to protect himself from the rain. The king's ministers eventually find his son and are shocked by his dirty, impoverished condition. They remind him of his true status as prince and future king of a vast kingdom and take him back to his joyful father.

Our birthright, according to Ayurveda, is to experience the full potential of life that comes only from living in complete conscious attunement with our universal nature. What is it then in the inherent nature of the mind that is capable of either strengthening or weakening this functional connection? The answer to this question has to do with the quality of the mind. We can better comprehend the meaning of this term, quality of mind, if we first understand the three qualities that govern physical existence.

All phenomena in the universe come under the influence of three primary phases of activity called the three *gunas*. Nature uses its creative mode, referred to as *sattva*, to bring life into manifestation. It then uses its organizing, activating phase, called *rajas*, to build and maintain what has just been created. When the purpose of that stage is complete, it uses its destructive mode, called *tamas*, to bring it to an end. The influence of these three *gunas* is universal and all-pervasive. Nothing in existence is outside their realm of influence.

What do these three phases of creation have to do with the mind? The same *gunas* that govern all existence also regulate our minds. As it manifests in the mind, *sattva* gives us the desire to know, as well as the capacity to create, to think and to imagine. It expresses itself as curiosity, fascination and inspiration. *Rajas* generates action, initiative and motivation, and expresses itself in the ability to organize and implement. *Tamas* in the mind supplies us with the ability to bring to completion whatever was created through *sattva* and produced through *rajas*.

The following example will help illustrate this point. Suppose that someone decides to build a house. *Sattva* allows them to picture living in a new house and what this new house would be like. They present their dream to an architect who then imagines all the details and creates drawings from which the house will be built. The *sattvic* property of *manas* allows the house to be conceived and designed down to the smallest detail. At this point the house exists in its completeness, but only in the mind of the architect.

Rajas now comes into play to make the architect's plans a physical reality. The plans are given to a builder, who coordinates all the activities of constructing the house with the subcontractors and laborers. These people then take various raw materials and organize them in the form of a house which conforms to the architect's design.

For the house to be completed, the creative thinking of *sattva* and the building activity of *rajas* must, at some point, come to a conclusion. This is the function of *tamas*. If the architect keeps showing up with creative new additions to the plans, or the builder keeps right on building, the house will never be completed. The original dream to have a new house can only be achieved when *tamas* brings the project to completion. Without the well-orchestrated coordination of all three *gunas*, the house could never be built.

Another common example is that of a little child who is given a new toy. Her curiosity, created by *sattva*, makes her want to discover and explore its possibilities. The *rajasic* quality of her mind motivates her to play with it, grab it, put it in her mouth, bang it and roll it around on the floor. Eventually, *tamas* will overwhelm the baby's natural curiosity, causing her to become bored with the toy and forget about it.

These examples demonstrate the beneficial role that each *guna* plays in the functioning of the mind. They do not, however, exist in equal proportion to one another. There is a natural, but disproportionate, parity among the three that keeps human life in optimum balance and moving in a positive, evolutionary direction.

The Proper Balance of the *Gunas*

Though we are all basically the same, our reactions to events and circumstances will differ widely. This is because our responses to life originate in the mind. How we respond depends, in part, on the specific balance of *sattva*, *rajas* and *tamas* in our minds.

What constitutes the proper balance of the *guna*s in the mind? This is directly reflected in the natural balance that exists among the *guna*s in creation. Life, in the broadest sense of the word, is essentially creative because the source from which everything springs is *param atma* — universal creative intelligence. Because of the intimate connection between *param atma* and *jiva atma*, the basic nature of the soul is also creative. This, in turn, directly influences the mind, causing it to be primarily creative or *sattvic*, with just enough *rajas* and *tamas* to bring desires into fruition. It is vital for health and happiness that the mind maintains this primarily creative influence in order to keep life always moving in a progressive direction.

What happens when this ideal proportion is not maintained? The following example will help illustrate what occurs when the mind is predominantly governed by a quality other than *sattva*. Imagine that fifty people are sitting in a hall and the fire alarm sounds. People with *rajas* dominating their mind will immediately jump up and begin to run around, searching for a fire extinguisher. This occurs because too much *rajas* creates a reliance on activity. Those with *tamas* dominating may panic and flee or faint because a predominance of *tamas* in the mind will create an influence of dullness, confusion and fearfulness. However, those people with a strong influence of *sattva* will calmly analyze the situation before acting, and attempt to create order in a potentially chaotic situation.

Of the three types listed above, most people would find the *sattva*-dominant mind to be the most desirable in a situation like this. *Sattva* lends itself toward calm, clear, creative thinking, a state of mind that allows one to easily find effective solutions to life's problems. The lesser qualities of *rajas* can then be relied upon to implement these solutions and *tamas* to bring these activities to an end when the problem has actually been solved. An influence of too much *rajas* or *tamas* can distort the naturally positive aspects of these supportive qualities and have a negative impact on our lives.

Excessive Influence of *Rajas* and *Tamas* on the Mind

It is the type of stimuli influencing the mind that causes the natural balance of the *guna*s to become distorted. These stimuli have three sources. The first is generated by the mind itself and has to do with the kind of thoughts and emotions on which we focus our attention. The second source has to do with the types of things we choose to take in through the senses. The final source of stimuli is the body, influencing *manas* through what we eat and drink. Of course, what we take in through the senses, as well as the type and quality of food we ingest, is a matter of choice and is ultimately determined by the mind.

Any stimulus, whether mental, sensory or physical, can have a predominantly *sattvic*, *rajasic* or *tamasic* influence on the mind. *Rajasic* stimuli include anything that keeps the mind in its active phase. In too great a quantity, these activating stimuli can prevent the mind from settling down. The mind then becomes unable to maintain its quiet, subtle connection with its source — *atma*, whose nature is peaceful, creative and limitlessly comprehensive.

This over-stimulated state of *manas* can be produced, for instance, by eating hot, spicy or fried foods; eating too many sweets; drinking liquids with caffeine or other stimulants; eating hurriedly or working and exercising too hard. Watching too much TV, action-oriented movies and loud, stimulating music can have a *rajasic* effect. Excessive thinking or feeling can also adversely influence the state of our minds.

A good example of behavior that can produce too much *rajas* in the mind is the lifestyle of the typical modern businessman. For many such people, breakfast may consist of a large cup of coffee and a donut gulped down on the way to the car. After fighting traffic all the way to work, he walks into the office to find an over-booked appointment schedule. For lunch he goes to a fast-food Mexican restaurant and eats hot, spicy food and drinks more coffee or caffeinated sodas. The afternoon consists of more appointments, meetings, pressured decisions and coffee, not to mention another hour-long battle with traffic on the ride home.

By the time this professional gets home, he feels quite agitated. Instead of being able to enjoy family life, he gets irritated by the little things his spouse or children do. He tries to read to divert his mind but he cannot concentrate. When it is time to go to bed, he finds that sleep will not come. His mind is still racing even though he feels exhausted. Continuously on the go and unable to stop even at night, the influence of *rajas* in his mind will continue to grow affecting both his health and happiness.

Too much stimuli of a *tamas*ic nature will produce heaviness, dullness or inertia in the mind. These qualities obscure the light of *atma* and its clear, creative, inspired nature. This lethargic state can be produced by eating foods that are aged, like cheese, or stale, like leftovers, eating too much red meat, drinking alcohol, taking drugs or becoming fatigued. Alcohol offers a clear example of the negative impact of *tamas*ic substances. A normally bright, clear, respectful individual will, through the use of alcohol, become confused, angry and disrespectful of others. Even after just one or two drinks, his mental and sensory functioning may slow and dim and the knowledge that he is acting inappropriately is obscured by the dulling influence of *tamas*.

The *sattvic* mind always chooses those things that promote growth and fulfillment, because the connection with its pure, creative source is always maintained. It is inherently aware of the things that are beneficial for it. When *rajas* dominates, however, the mind becomes unsteady, and even though it has the knowledge of what is best, it will often stray from doing those things. When *tamas* dominates, the mind forgets what is good for it, and becomes lost in thoughts and actions which have negative or destructive effects.

To repeat this very important point, it is in the improper functioning of the mind that the seeds of disease are sown. If *manas* loses the influence of *sattva*, it loses conscious contact with the limitless power of *atma* that is naturally available to it. Without the full support of nature's intelligence and organizing power, life no longer proceeds spontaneously in an evolutionary direction.

As a result of this, individuals become frustrated in their ability to fulfill their desires. They become less efficient than they could be and find themselves working harder but accomplishing less. Clarity, inspiration and motivation decrease, fatigue increases, and dependency on *rajas*ic and *tamas*ic stimuli grows in order to artificially enhance the functioning of the mind, senses and body. This imbalance then leads the mind to make further harmful choices, creating a destructive spiral away from health and happiness. Human life then becomes like an anchorless, rudderless ship set adrift on a stormy ocean.

Ayurveda's gift is the removal of the *tamas* or ignorance which clouds the mind and causes us to lose sight of our universal status. This is accomplished not only by eliminating the toxic impurities from the body, but by educating the individual to never allow these imbalances to occur in the first place. What we eat and what we do play a very important role in who we are.

Effects of Diet and Lifestyle on the Mind

Ayurveda often demonstrates the concept of "who we are is influenced by what we eat" in the example of the elephant, the tiger and the jackal. The elephant is a *sattvic* animal that eats only fresh, vegetarian food. It is large, strong and gentle, and because of its intelligence, learns to work well with human beings. The tiger exemplifies *rajas*. He kills and eats the flesh of other animals. He has a fierce, aggressive nature but is very restless and is always on the prowl. The jackal shows the less desirable qualities of *tamas*. Rather than seek its own food, it eats whatever is left over after another animal has eaten. It tends to be a fearful and lazy animal that is nocturnal and shuns daylight.

When people ask what they can do to get control of their minds and emotions and become more positive in their outlook, I encourage them to look to their diet and lifestyle. I ask them what they are doing in their daily routine to increase *sattva* in their minds? Are they meditating daily and doing *yoga asanas* and *pranayam*? Are they eating a *sattvic* diet, keeping the company of the wise, and engaging in those activities that are conducive to positivity and joy? These are the things that help maintain a strong *sattvic* balance in the mind. Chapter Six of this book is devoted to the Ayurvedic understanding of diet and lifestyle choices that help us re-establish and maintain our eternal connection to *atma*. Metaphorically speaking, the wave then rediscovers that it is, and always was, nothing but the ocean.

Since the behaviors and reactions that support or undermine our health, happiness and wholeness originate in *manas*, an Ayurvedic physician will always begin his examination with an assessment of the patient's state of mind. The patient's attitude toward their healing process is often a good indication of the particular quality that dominates their mind.

Patients with a *sattvic* nature come to a physician with a cooperative and relaxed attitude. They describe their symptoms calmly and clearly and can be counted on to follow the physician's instructions. They are curious about their illness and how their body functions and try to understand why they have fallen ill. People with *sattvic* minds usually take responsibility for their own health and prefer not to rely too heavily on doctors or medicines.

Patients with more *rajas* exaggerate their symptoms with an air of impatience and desperation. They tend to become dependent on doctors and medicines for their health and may hop from specialist to specialist seeking relief. They will often follow the physician's advice so meticulously that they may make frequent calls to clarify details.

Individuals with *tamas*ic minds will often not be able to describe their symptoms clearly. They may show confusion or be less cooperative and may forget or somehow not be able to follow the physician's instructions. In essence, they are too dull to effectively discern and follow the path back to health.

Dhi, Dhruti and *Smriti*

Once the physician has assessed the nature of a patient's mind, he can design a suitable treatment for the patient. The physician's treatment always attempts to increase *sattva* so the person can return to a state where they inherently know what is good for them. Ayurveda calls this knowingness, *dhi*. He also tries to increase *dhruti*, the more life-supporting aspect of *rajas*, which motivates the patient to actually do the things he knows to be good for him, i.e., follow the physician's instructions. Finally, the physician works to enliven the quality of *smriti* in the patient's awareness. *Smriti* is associated with the beneficial function of *tamas*, and causes the patient to stop unhealthy activities and remember the healthy ones.

An example of these three positive functions of *manas* is shown in the case of wanting to stop smoking cigarettes. *Dhi* tells me that smoking is injurious to my health. *Dhruti* causes me to avoid reaching for a cigarette. If I do occasionally lapse and have a smoke, *smriti* reminds me of the importance of abstaining from cigarettes. Because of the critical function of *manas* in life and health, it is essential to enhance these beneficial qualities of the mind.

INDRIYA: THE FIVE SENSES

The *indriyas*, or senses, are the third major component of life described by Ayurveda. They arise out of the fundamental properties inherent in the five elements, a process which will be explained in detail in the next chapter. The *indriyas* act as a bridge between the non-physical parts of life: *atma* or soul and the mind on one side, and the physical body and environment on the other. Without the senses, our internal reality would be completely disconnected from our external reality.

The *indriyas* gather information from the outer world. Incoming perceptions get relayed to the mind in the form of sound; touch and temperature; light, color and form; taste and flavor; and smell. If the perceptual information gathered by the senses is of proper quality and quantity, it will have an uplifting and supporting influence on the mind. If it is not, it will create imbalance in the mind and, eventually, imbalance in the body.

After loss of knowingness, which Ayurveda calls *pragya aparadha*, it states that the primary cause of disease is the improper use of the senses with their objects. The Sanskrit term for this is *asatmya-indriyartha-samyog*. Misuse of the senses can occur in three ways. First, we can take in excessive sensory stimuli. This can occur by listening to music that is too loud, living in noisy environs, watching too much TV or working long hours at the computer. Talking excessively or reading too much can also overload the senses.

Insufficient sensory input constitutes the second way to misuse the senses and includes all situations where there is a deficit of sensory perception. Seasonal Affect Disorder offers a clear example. This syndrome occurs in extreme northern climates during the winter months when there is very little sunlight available, and causes affective disorders such as depression. Another example is the isolation of solitary confinement, such as would occur in prisons or prisoner-of-war camps. It is well known that such situations can cause great agitation and mental imbalance in prisoners.

Sensory intake which is morally or emotionally repugnant represents the third misuse of the senses. Seeing or hearing things which are distressing can disrupt the balance between mind and body. Movies and television, for instance, with their constant emphasis on physical and emotional violence, fill the airwaves with strong sensory impressions that impact the nervous system adversely. Misuse not only impairs the senses themselves, weakening the coordination between the mind and body which they serve, but directly harms the mind and damages the body.

The Differences Between Senses and Organs of Sense

At this point, it is useful to make a distinction between the senses and the organs of perception through which these senses function. Unlike the physical sense organs, the senses themselves have no material reality, but rather are subtle, subjective processes. The process of perception involves a movement from the external, material objects of perception, through the physical organs of sense, to the senses themselves. This constitutes a movement from the gross to subtle, from concrete to abstract.

Senses and Organs of Perception and Five Elements

SENSE	ORGAN OF PERCEPTION	ELEMENT
Hearing	Ear	Akash
Touch	Skin	Vayu
Sight	Eye	Agni
Taste	Tongue	Jala
Smell	Nose	Prithvi

The organ of sight (the eye) is able to perceive because there is the sense of sight present and functioning through it. The sense of sight, on the other hand, doesn't require a physical organ in order to function. When a sense organ is no longer present or properly functioning, what is lost is not the sense itself, but the sense's usual vehicle for connecting with the outside world. This is true for all five senses and their respective organs.

To clarify this distinction, let's examine the physical organ of sight. The eye sees when the sense of sight functions through it. However, when the sense of sight is absent, as in deep sleep or a coma, even a physically perfect eye is unable to see. On the other hand, the sense of sight is lively and active even when the organ of sight is not functioning, as in the case of an inner vision or a dream, where we are "seeing" something in our "mind's eye." This inner perception can happen with our eyes closed, or in the dark with no light whatsoever striking the eye. The sense of sight is still functioning but on a much subtler level than we normally associate with it.

Each sense and its corresponding organ of perception are highly specialized. They perform a function that no other sense or sense organ nor any other part of the body can do. Only the eye can see; only the ear can hear, etc.

The Protective Nature of the Senses

The senses carry information from the outside to the inside and back again with remarkable ease and speed. When we eat incorrectly and get indigestion, the senses bring information about the body's digestive distress to the mind's attention. The mind can then decide not to eat again until the stomach settles down.

A child playing in the back yard hears a sound. Based on the information which the senses bring to her attention, she can distinguish between the threatening bark of a dog and the comforting sound of her mother's voice. Even animals, which do not have the developed intellect of human beings, can discriminate between the environment's life-supporting and nourishing influences and its toxic and harmful ones.

Proper functioning of the *indriyas* is crucial to the maintenance of good health. Fortunately, there is an inherent intelligence within each sense that tries to protect the mind and body from too much, too little or the improper kind of sensory impressions. For example, if the lights are too bright, we will automatically shield our eyes; if the music is too loud or too soft, we will get up and adjust the volume. As little children, before we became "desensitized," if we saw a scary scene in a movie, we would close or cover our eyes.

The senses, when alert, connected and used correctly, are essential to the process of making choices which create and maintain health. To determine the quality of sensory functioning, we must look at the effects of both body and mind on the senses. Physical disease can impact sensory perception by compromising the operation of the sense organs. When we have a cold, both our nose and ears get congested, inhibiting our ability to hear, taste and smell things in our environment.

The Adverse Impact of the Mind on the Senses

A *rajasic* mind may constantly choose sensory input which damages the organs of perception, such as loud music which stresses the hearing mechanism. In addition to the impact on our sensory apparatus, the quality of mind also determines the caliber of perception. A *tamasic* mind actually dulls the receptive capacity of the senses, which then transmit distorted or incomplete information about the body and environment. Alcohol, for instance, deadens the senses. Consequently, we have laws against driving while intoxicated.

With a *sattvic* mind, the senses are finely tuned receptors and highly accurate transmitters of information to and from the body and environment. Guided by the soul, the *sattvic* mind selects things which protect, nourish and strengthen the parts of life and their connections. Ayurveda sees this vital, integrated mode of functioning as the basis of health and happiness.

Since the *indriyas* are the link between ourselves and the outside world, it is important to understand from where these non-material sensory capacities originate. The next chapter examines the relationship between the five senses and the five elements.

SHARIRA: THE BODY

Sharira, the body, is the fourth fundamental part of life. Ayurveda does not consider *sharira* to be any more important than the subtler parts of human life just described. It does, however, understand the body to be the vehicle through which we can influence these aspects and their connections with each other and the whole. The next several chapters are devoted to the Ayurvedic conception of the human body and the principles which govern its functioning.

V

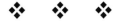

Chapter Two

PANCHAMAHABHUTA: THE FIVE ELEMENT THEORY

*T*he last aspect of human life to be elaborated is *sharira*, the physical body. When viewed in its proper perspective, the body is nothing less than an evolutionary wonder, an unbelievably complex instrument capable of supporting limitless possibilities for human life. This marvel of nature can be studied from many points of view. Our Western model has taught us to see the body as a thing or object composed of successively smaller objects: organs, cells, organelles, molecules, atoms and sub-atomic particles.

Though Ayurveda does not argue the validity of this "objective" view of the body, it takes a somewhat different perspective. Rather than place so much emphasis on the strictly material nature of the body's components, it maintains that it is far more useful to understand the underlying principles that order and govern their functioning. The same dynamics that orchestrate the processes within the human body also orchestrate life everywhere in the universe. The conceptual model that Ayurveda uses to understand the principles of nature's functioning is called *Panchamahabhuta* or the theory of the five great elements.

This theory serves as the foundation for all of Ayurveda's diagnostic and treatment modalities and has allowed physicians for thousands of years to successfully detect and treat imbalances anywhere in human life. *Charaka Samhita*, the primary Ayurvedic text, states: "One must master the understanding of the elements in order to be a physician." While considerable training and experience is required to turn this knowledge into clinical skill, a general grasp of it will offer a practical and therapeutically useful comprehension of the vital interrelationship between man and nature.

The basic premise of the *Panchamahabhuta* theory is that everything in physical creation is composed of five fundamental building blocks of nature called elements. In the West, most people are familiar with only four elements, the ones commonly known as earth, air, fire and water. However, Ayurveda recognizes the element of space to be the first and most basic of the five elements. These *bhutas* or elements are understood to be the most fundamental properties of physical creation.

Since the five elements fall within the realm of material, observable creation and can be objectively studied, it is curious that modern science has overlooked their utility in understanding both the human body and physical existence in general. The reason for this is twofold. First, as modern science became more and more object-oriented in its approach to studying life, it became less process-oriented. As a result, it has failed to develop a sufficiently comprehensive understanding of the underlying principles that govern the world of objects. Because of their abstract and invisible nature, these "laws of nature" are difficult to be objectified.

But just because we cannot "see" the local, state and national laws which govern society's interactions, doesn't mean that their influence does not exist. When we visit a foreign land, we can deduce from peoples' actions the codes of conduct that regulate them. Ayurveda takes a similar, subjective approach to understanding the existence of these unseen laws of nature's functioning.

Ayurveda calls these universal organizing principles *mahabhutas*, or cosmic elements. They are the essence or inherent intelligence within each *bhuta* or element, which allows it to function with the specific qualities and characteristics that are unique to it. Unlike the *bhutas*, the *mahabhutas* have no dimension, no states and no physical properties. In the process of the creation unfolding from universal intelligence, the *mahabhutas* precede the *bhutas* and are more fundamental and comprehensive in their scope.

It is not possible to comprehend the nature of the elements as basic building blocks of physical creation without understanding their underlying organizing principles. It is this knowledge that defines the function of the *bhutas*, and thus gives the five element theory its practical utility for understanding the body.

Because modern science lacks this more comprehensive understanding of nature, it has failed to see the connection between the processes that happen in the universe at large and those that occur within the human body. For thousands of years, Ayurveda has observed that the same laws of nature which govern the elements and their interactions in the world must necessarily govern the elements within our bodies. Our bodies are structured from the food we eat, the water we drink and the air we breathe. These things are nothing but the various combinations of the five elements. Therefore, how could our physical nature be anything but the elements? There is no difference, we are part and parcel with nature!

The Elements and Their Sequence of Manifestation

In Ayurveda, the five elements of space, air, fire, water and earth and their corresponding organizing principles are termed respectively: *akash*, *vayu*, *agni*, *jala* and *prithvi*. In this book, we will favor the Sanskrit names because the common English terms do not accurately convey the true meaning of these principles. When we do use the terms air, fire, water, etc., understand that they are used in a figurative sense and are rarely meant to be taken literally. To do so tends to limit our ability to understand the utility of the five element theory.

The ancient Ayurvedic texts describe the way physical creation manifests as an orderly, sequential unfoldment of the *bhutas*. The elements do not physically manifest all at once. Rather, they come into existence in the same way that life unfolds—from the most subtle and comprehensive values to the most material, limited values. Each preceding element is subtler in nature and serves as a foundation for the manifestation of each succeeding element.

Sequential Flow of Elements

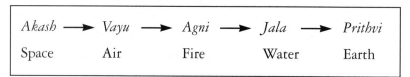

Akash	Vayu	Agni	Jala	Prithvi
Space	Air	Fire	Water	Earth

Thus, the first element to come into physical existence is *akash* or space. Of the five elements, *akash* has the most expansive, least concrete value. The next element to manifest is *vayu*, commonly referred to as air. It has a more tangible quality than *akash* but not as much as *agni*, the fire element. The last elements to manifest in the sequence are *jala* or water and finally *prithvi*, the earth element. These elements are clearly more concrete or material than their predecessors. The logic of the bhuta's sequential emergence will become clear as we observe specific processes by which nature manifests physical creation.

To understand how the ancient Ayurvedic scientist used observation of natural events to deduce the existence of the *mahabhutas*, let's look at a seed and the processes which it undergoes to become a tree. A seed is normally hard and compact. When we put it between our fingers and squeeze it, we notice that it is difficult to compress because of its density. However, once the sprouting process begins, the seed grows less dense as it starts to expand. This expansion takes place in all directions simultaneously. We can now compress the seed and it no longer offers resistance to our pressure. These qualities of nonresistance and uni-directional expansion typify the element of *akash*. It exists because the quality of spaciousness is growing in the seed and there is proportionately less matter to offer resistance. Spaciousness is necessary in order for any further development to take place, so *akash* dominates the first stage of growth in any life form.

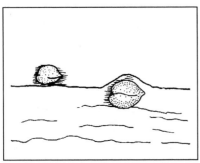

Seed in its *Akash* manifestation

Next we notice that the expansion which was occurring in all directions starts to take a specific course. Inside the seed, a sprout begins to form. Cell multiplication now takes a particular orientation. This uni–directional movement is due to a single, propulsive force exerting itself upon the seed, much like the wind exerts its directive action upon a leaf. This force comes from the element of *vayu*, the principle in creation which governs movement and direction.

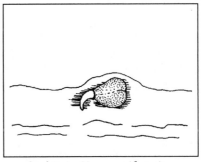

Seed in its *Vayu* manifestation

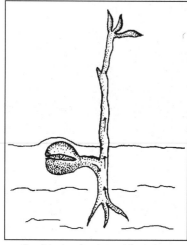

Seed in its *Agni* manifestation

In order for the sprout to break free of its casing and grow out through the earth into the open air, there now has to be a metabolic breakdown of the outer shell. To achieve this, the seed begins to increase thermogenesis. This change in temperature results from a change in the seed's pH value which is caused by acid–alkaline conversion. *Agni* controls this stage of the growth process. Even though *agni* is called the fire element, there is no actual fire that takes place within the seed but there is some increase in heat that enables the metabolic transformation to occur.

Jala bhuta, the water element, accomplishes the seed's fourth stage of growth. As metabolism continues, a need arises to transport nutrients from the seed to the growing sprout. The principle of *jala* governs liquefaction, cohesion and the growth mechanism through which the plant adds to itself, unit by unit.

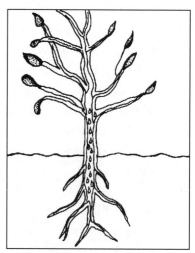

Seed in its *Jala* manifestation)

Eventually, the predominantly liquid form of the plant starts to acquire more shape and structure. Minerals flow to the various parts of the plant and get consolidated into particular forms unique to it: the structures that eventually will manifest as branches, leaves, etc. The dominance of *prithvi* or the earth element, governs this stage of the seed's evolution. Each succeeding stage of growth incorporates the elements which have influenced the previous stages. By the

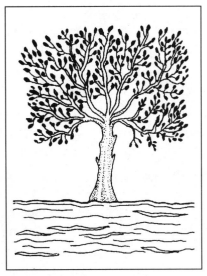

Seed in its *Prithvi* manifestation

time we see *prithvi* bhuta creating form in the plant, the other four elements are working in close coordination with it.

Human life develops in the exact same way under the influence of the five elements. After insemination, the fertilized ovum, called a blastula, starts immediately to multiply itself. In the beginning, this cell multiplication occurs in a symmetric, omni–directional manner. Within a short period of time, however, the symmetry breaks and the expansion acquires a longitudinal direction, as well as a differentiation of layers that takes place from the inside out.

Up to this point, cell multiplication has been fed by nutrients supplied by the parental material (ovum and sperm). However, at the stage where cell multiplication takes a direction, there is need for a new energy source. The blastula must now start to convert the raw materials supplied by the mother through the umbilical cord into its own nutrients. This is the stage at which metabolic conversion begins. The nutrients created by this conversion process are then bound up in a liquid medium and transported to the various layers (derms) and regions of growth differentiation. This liquid flow of nutrients allows the fetus to increase in size. At this point, the fetus has a primarily liquid form. After about the third month, however, it begins to take on a more defined shape and structure. That is why ultrasound cannot be used to diagnose specific abnormalities in fetal formation until after the third month.

These examples help to demonstrate the influence of the *mahabhutas* and how they orchestrate the sequential unfoldment of the five elements in the formation of life. This specific sequence of manifestation is invariable. The last developmental stage, typified by form and structure, will never occur before the organizing intelligences previous to it have accomplished their purpose.

A more in-depth analysis of the inherent qualities of each element will help us to fully grasp the significance of the five element theory in understanding the human body. In addition, it will assist us in comprehending the nature of the *indriyas* or senses because it is from the elements that the senses and their respective sense organs arise.

AKASH: THE PRINCIPLE OF SPACE

Akash (Space) and its Qualities

Akash (Space)	Non-Resistance Sound

When we think of deep space, we imagine an incomprehensibly vast expanse of open, unobstructed nothingness. Yet, within this "no-thing-ness" is contained the possibility for things or objects to be present. This no-thing-ness is the element of space, and without it, nothing in the universe can exist nor can any process take place. *Akash*, the subtlest of the *bhutas*, serves as a matrix or medium in which the other *bhutas* can manifest. Objects in creation exist in relationship to one another by virtue of space. Space creates the relationship and allows us to have knowledge of things within our perceptual field. Because the essential nature of *akash* is free of objects, non-resistance is one of its basic properties. Nothing exists to offer resistance when *akash* is found by itself.

Sound

After non-resistance, sound is the second fundamental quality of *akash*. We know that sound propagates by virtue of space. What is not so apparent is that sound is actually born out of the creation of space. Whenever there is a sudden separation between any particles or objects that have been bound together, sound occurs. Take, for example, a piece of chalk. When we break a stick of chalk, we hear a snap; when we write on the board with it, we hear a scraping sound. In both cases, particles of chalk are abruptly being separated from each other; i.e., space is suddenly being created between them. A few more examples will help illustrate this principle.

When we blow up a balloon, we pressurize or compress the particles of air inside. If, instead of tying off the balloon, we allow the air to escape, we will hear a flapping, gushing noise, due to a sudden expansion of the space between the air particles as it is released from the balloon.

When we talk, we send pressurized air across the vocal cords and through the mouth cavity. Variations in the tension of these folds of tissue and the shape of the mouth change the capacity of the air particles to expand or separate from one another. The many different sounds which the voice produces are dependent on precise modulations of the space within the throat and mouth.

A carpenter uses sound to evaluate the quality of a piece of wood by knocking on it to determine its density or porosity. The more open and resonant the sound, the more space he knows exists between the fibers of wood, and therefore, the less structurally sound it is. He will reject that piece of wood in favor of one that has a duller sound to it. Again, greater mass creates greater resistance to sound. Similarly, a carpenter can find the wooden supports in a wall by knocking on it in various places and listening for where the dull, thudding sounds occur.

A close relationship exists between each *bhuta* and sense organ, and *akash*'s corresponding sense organ is the ear. The ear is a hollow, spacious structure containing very thin, light bones—the smallest, most porous bones in the body—and is responsible for translating sound from the environment into neural impulses. *Akash*'s predominance in the structure of the organ of hearing is responsible for the production of sound.

VAYU: THE PRICIPLE OF MOVEMENT, DRYING AND SEPARATION

Vayu (Air) and its Qualities

Vayu (Air)	Movement Touch

In popular discussions of five-element theory, the element of *vayu* is often translated as air or wind, but this is only a figurative interpretation. The Ayurvedic classics clearly explain that movement is the essential organizing principle behind this *bhuta*. Since movement always implies direction, these two qualities are closely associated. *Vayu* originates and gives direction to all motion and change, and, as a result, to all processes and functions in creation.

This principle governs the movement of everything in the universe, from the tiniest subatomic particles to the most immense, swirling galaxies. It gives the wind its direction. It causes the earth to quake and volcanoes to spew fire. *Vayu* impels blood to flow through our veins, food to move through our intestinal tracts and neural impulses to be carried at lightning speeds to and from our brains.

Movement also generates a drying influence, which in turn produces separation or disintegration, another important aspect of *vayu*. This will be more clearly understood when we discuss the elements of *jala* and *prithvi*.

The Sense of Touch

Just as the sense of hearing is intimately associated with the principle of *akash*, the sense of touch arises out of the principle of movement or *vayu*. The skin, functioning as the organ of touch, is capable of detecting movement in the form of subtle or gross changes in pressure, friction or vibration. Movement against the skin can be registered as hard or soft, rough or smooth, blunt or sharp and fast or slow. This information is encoded in neural impulses and transmitted to the brain to be interpreted by the mind as good or bad, something to be enjoyed or avoided.

The following examples show the intimate connection between the sense of touch and the principle of movement. When a friend rests his hand lightly on your arm, you perceive his touch because you suddenly experience a difference in the pressure against your skin. If his hand doesn't move, you will soon forget that he is touching you. Any movement on his part will again remind you that his hand is there.

If you sit perfectly still in hot water, you stop feeling the wetness and warmth of water against your skin until you move again, stirring it into motion. The same is true for the clothes you wear. When you first put on a shirt, you feel it by virtue of the movement of the cloth against your skin. However, if you remain motionless for a time, the lack of friction causes you to forget about the shirt. Either the skin has to undergo movement or whatever contacts the skin must move. Without movement, there is no sense of touch; it is the difference in movement that produces the sense of touch.

Just as the element of *akash* governs those organs in the body that require space to function, *vayu* governs the organs whose functioning requires movement in the form of contraction and dilation, especially the colon, uterus and urinary bladder. The heart, with its constant pumping action, is also a major organ of *vayu*. Muscular movement, the blinking of the eyes, the transmission of nervous impulses to and from the brain——all happen as a result of *vayu*.

AGNI: THE PRINCIPLE OF COVERSION, HEAT AND LIGHT

Agni (Fire) and its Qualities

Agni	Coversion
(Fire)	Sight

Though popularly known as the fire element, *agni*'s essence is displayed in creation in many more ways than just the physical form of fire. *Agni*'s nature is best understood in terms of its universal organizing principle: the intelligence which causes all conversion or transformation in creation. This manifests as the qualities of heat and light, as well as that which gives color and visual form to all things.

Agni is third in the sequence of elements to manifest from cosmic intelligence. Just as *vayu* (motion) can only take place within the medium of *akash* (space), light and heat are produced from the pressure and friction inherent in movement. We can see this when we rub two sticks together to start a campfire. The sun offers perhaps the most striking example of this principle. As a result of the immense pressures that exist within the core of the sun, a nuclear reaction takes place, which generates emissions of radiant heat and photons of light. The light and heat which our planet receives from the sun constitute the primary source for all transformations. Sunlight acts as a catalyst in the production of carbohydrates in the chlorophyll-containing tissues of plants. The sun's heat, which warms the earth, is directly and indirectly responsible for all metabolic processes. Without it, there would be no transformations and, therefore, no life.

Conversion is the key concept in defining *agni*'s role in creation. In non-living systems, it is responsible for changing matter into increasingly entropic or decayed states; in living systems, it facilitates all growth processes. Fire is the most obvious manifestation of *agni*'s capacity to convert. When applied to a log, fire soon transforms it into carbon ash. When applied to food, it transforms cellular tissue into something easier for the body to assimilate.

Agni also supports change in less obvious ways. It stimulates conversion in both organic and inorganic processes through such things as catalysts, which affect or determine the rates of all chemical reactions; acids, which dissolve or break down chemical or biochemical bonds; and enzymes, which bring about or accelerate reactions at body temperatures. Even slight or moderate heat can produce transformations. Refrigerators retard the natural conversion process which would soon spoil food and milk at room temperature. In the form of light, *agni* generates photosynthesis in plants and changes darkness into visible colors and shapes.

In the human body, *agni bhuta* works in several different ways. Food metabolism, which Ayurveda figuratively calls "digestive fire," is the most obvious. No actual fire burns in the stomach and small intestine, but various acids and enzymes are secreted which cause a metabolic breakdown in the food we eat. The thermogenic effect of these secretions can be clearly experienced in the "burning" of hyperacidity.

On a subtler level, *agni*'s strength or weakness can be seen or felt in a person's radiance. The luster of a person's skin and the color of his complexion reflect the quality of light inherent in this element. Healthy people shine and project dynamism, while those in poor health appear lack-luster and dull. We can detect *agni* in the brilliance of the eyes. Contrast the glow in the eyes of a healthy, happy individual with the total lack of light coming from the eyes of someone who is deceased. Even though the body of a dead person has the same optic nerve, lens and pupil as the body of someone who is alive, the light in the eye is absent, because the connection with the cosmic aspect of *agni*, the "fire of life," has been extinguished.

The Sense of Sight

Our sense of sight is intimately associated with the element of *agni*. If it were not for *agni* in the form of light, creation would exist in amorphous darkness. Not only does *agni* allow us to see form and degrees of dark and light, it also allows us to see color. Everything that is illuminated reflects a different wavelength of light, which gives that object a unique color. Through the sense of sight, the eye takes in physical shape and color, to which the mind then ascribes a meaning.

JALA: THE PRINCIPLE OF LIQUIDITY AND COHESION

Jala (Water) and its Qualities

Jala (Water)	Liquidity Taste

Jala, the fourth element to arise sequentially from cosmic intelligence, is often translated as "water." Though water is of key importance to life on earth, it is imprecise to call it one of Ayurveda's five elements. As with the other elements, *jala*'s universal organizing principle, or *mahabhuta*, offers a more complete picture. When we understand the *mahabhuta* of *jala*, we know that it embodies the principle of liquidity and cohesion. In organic life, *jala* is also responsible for increasing size, since water is the primary constituent of all living forms.

Jala mahabhuta governs fluidity, irrespective of the substance or what is suspended in it. It governs a substance's ability to change shape without separating or losing its integrity. This integrity exists because of *jala*'s nature to bind or hold together. Even solid matter can demonstrate *jala*'s cohesive influence. If we pick up a dry, parched clod of earth, it will quickly and easily disintegrate and turn into dust. However, if there is moisture in the soil, the dirt particles in the lump of earth will remain bound together.

Though water provides the best example of *jala*'s properties of fluidity and cohesion, there are many other substances which display these qualities, yet contain little or no water. For instance, both volcanic lava and gasoline can flow and move freely and though they do not have a shape of their own, they maintain their integrity while taking on the form of that which contains them or through which they flow. This is seen with liquid in a glass, the blood in our veins, or water in a pond.

Water, the most common manifestation of *jala bhuta* on this planet, is the major component of all life forms. In the sap of a plant or tree, water acts as a medium through which *vayu* carries nutrients to leaves and branches. In blood, it performs the same function, binding nutrients and oxygen within itself so that *vayu* can move them throughout the body. As saliva and digestive secretions, it binds together nutrients which have been broken down by the transformative action of *agni*, and allows them to be carried by *vayu* through the G-I tract to further stages of digestion and elimination. *Jala* protects the mucous membranes of the body and lubricates the joints so that solid structures can move or flow more freely over one another. In the form of cerebrospinal fluid, it surrounds and protects the delicate nervous tissue of the brain and spinal cord.

The Sense of Taste

According to Ayurveda, the sense of taste arises out of *jala bhuta*. The ability to taste is dependent on the liquidity that exists within the mouth in the form of saliva. Imagine trying to taste something, much less swallow it, if your tongue and mouth are completely dry. Taste does not exist in a mouth totally devoid of moisture. Taste also does not occur when water is the only liquid in the mouth, since pure water is experienced by the sense of taste as an absolute — totally devoid of taste.

Jala, in the form of water or saliva, acts as a medium in which the sense of taste discerns the relative quality and quantity of solids dispersed within it. The body needs to know the proportion of solids to liquids, and the sense of taste gives the knowledge of how much solid content is contained in the substances we put into our mouths, as well as the composition of those substances.

When we are served a cup of tea, the sense of taste identifies the particles of tea suspended in the water, and determines the relative proportion of sweet flavor provided by the sugar to offset the tea's somewhat bitter flavor.

As we will discuss later, taste is a very important factor in both diet and digestion. Ayurveda describes six fundamental tastes or flavors that are found in food: Sweet, sour, salty, bitter, pungent and astringent. These tastes arise out of the varying predominance of the five elements that compose that food substance. The human body is also composed of all five elements, but some elements exist in greater proportion than others.

The body has an innate wisdom regarding food selection, which functions through the sense of taste. The body favors those foods that reflect its specific elemental make-up. The sense of taste gives us an indication of the elemental make-up of food and thereby protects us from ingesting substances that may upset the natural balance of the elements in our body. This explains why, when we are offered unfamiliar food, we will first sample only a small amount on the tip of a spoon or finger before taking a larger amount. It also explains why we are more inclined to eat a bowl of fruit or sweetened cereal than a bowl of cayenne pepper. The body contains relatively small amounts of *agni* and large amounts of *jala*. Sweet flavors are more readily accepted by the body because they are closely associated with the water element. To ingest a large amount of *agni* in the form of cayenne pepper would greatly disturb the natural balance of the elements in the body.

The tongue is extremely well-suited to be an organ of taste. Full and fleshy, its construction allows maximum surface contact with the watery element that constantly surrounds it. Through the tongue the sensory mechanism judges the appropriate tastes and quantities to be ingested, thus protecting the body and helping to keep it in balance.

PRITHVI: THE PRICIPLE OF FORM AND STRUCTURE

Prithvi (Earth) and its Qualities

Prithvi (Earth)	Solidity Smell

The sequential manifestation of the elements moves from subtle and abstract to gross and concrete. Consequently, *prithvi* or "earth," the most solid of the elements, is the last to emerge. Solidity and structure describe the essence of the cosmic organizing principle for this element. Any substance or particle with shape, no matter what its size, indicates the presence of *prithvi bhuta*. All structure, whether in an atom, a molecule, a rock, a mountain, a planet, a solar system or a galaxy, is determined by *prithvi*. This element governs the shape and structure of every branch, leaf and flower in the plant kingdom and every organ, tendon, muscle and bone in the animal kingdom.

The Sense of Smell

Prithvi bhuta is closely associated with the sense of smell, and a brief analysis will demonstrate their connection. Whenever *vayu*'s drying influence removes the cohesion supplied to a substance by *jala*, nothing keeps the particles of matter in that substance bound together, regardless of whether the substance is a solid, semi-solid, liquid or gas. Tiny particles begin to separate out from the substance and *vayu* disperses them in all directions. They eventually come in contact with the nose, the organ of smell. Each of the scattered, microscopic bits of matter has its own chemical signature, i.e., its own molecular shape or structure, which the olfactory mechanism is able to recognize. The mind interprets this sensory information as a specific smell.

Any substance with abundant water will not have as strong a smell as something dry. Take, for instance, coriander seeds. In seed form coriander has only a faint scent. However, when the seeds are crushed, the particles separate from each other and encounter increased exposure to *vayu*. When the moisture content decreases and *jala* can no longer hold the chemical structure together, we begin to experience coriander's sweet smell. If the spice is heated, causing even more water to evaporate, a powerful fragrance will be diffused throughout the room.

The sense of smell can give us information about an object or substance, without having to see its full shape or mass. If someone leaves a fish on the kitchen counter for a brief period, the drying influence of *vayu* minimizes *jala*'s cohesive function. *Prithvi bhuta*, in the form of tiny particles of fish, will then disperse throughout the kitchen. Our sense of smell will be able to recognize the odor long after the fish has been put back into the freezer. Whenever an odor is detected, *prithvi* is there. In the absence of detectable smell, *prithvi*'s presence can be determined by the hardness and shape of things.

Prithvi, like the other elements, serves a protective function by preventing us from taking in anything harmful. When our sense of smell detects noxious fumes, we quickly turn away. When presented with unfamiliar food, we often sniff it first before deciding whether to eat it. We are naturally attracted to fresh, sweet smells and repulsed by stale, putrid odors. Ayurveda recognizes that smells, like tastes, have a predictable effect on the balance of the *bhutas* in the physiology, and uses aroma therapy as one of its treatment modalities.

The structure of each sense organ reflects the quality of the element from which the sense arises. The nose, therefore, has a hard composition. It protrudes from the plane of the face to facilitate receiving the particles of *prithvi* floating in the air.

In conclusion, if we compare the qualities of the elements with the structure of their corresponding sense organs, we can also gain confirmation of the relationship between the *bhutas* or elements and the senses. The organ of hearing, the ear, is a hollow, structure with extremely light and porous bones, reflecting *akash's* quality of spaciousness. The skin, the organ of touch, is the driest, thinnest and most sensitive organ of the body, corresponding to *vayu's* ability to react to the smallest movement. The eye is the only organ in the body that actually has a brilliance or shine emanating from it, mirroring *agni's* light. The tongue, the organ of taste, is covered by watery secretions and discerns dissolved solids, reflecting *jala's* fluid and cohesive nature. Lastly, the nose, the organ of smell, is more solid than the other sense organs. It is structured to receive fine particles and molecules, and shows *prithvi's* tendency for mass and form.

Diagnostic Utility of the Elements and Their Senses

The concept of the five universal elements, their corresponding physical elements and the senses that arise from them, provides a broad framework for understanding how nature operates in the universe as a whole and within the human body. The practical application of this knowledge provides a clear window into mental and physiological functioning. It allows the Ayurvedic physician to use his senses to perform a thorough and accurate diagnosis, avoiding more costly or invasive procedures.

He uses his knowledge of how each sense derives from the qualities of its originating element. Sound cannot exist without space and lack of resistance, qualities of *akash*; touch depends on vibration or movement, aspects of *vayu*; sight occurs because of light and heat, characteristics of *agni*; taste cannot function without the liquid and cohesive nature of *jala*; and smell needs *prithvi's* solidity and form.

The physician knows that a sense's intimacy with its *bhuta* makes it the best vehicle to inform him of the presence and the state of that particular element in the body. The five *bhutas* have a natural balance in the body. *Jala* and *prithvi* normally predominate, whereas the others, because of their more powerful influence, are found only in microform. They all work in precise and balanced coordination with one another. This natural balance, however, can be disturbed by a number of different influences which we will elaborate on in later chapters.

Ayurveda employs a number of different diagnostic techniques using the senses to detect imbalances in the elements within the body. Auscultation, or thumping the body's various cavities, is used to give the physician knowledge of the functioning of the presence or lack of *akash* or space. For instance, the resonance will tell him if there is an atrophied organ or the opposite, a tumorous growth.

Perhaps the most versatile of all the senses for diagnostic purposes is the sense of touch. It not only gives knowledge of that element's functioning but can inform the physician of the state of the other four elements in the body. *Nadi vigyan* or pulse diagnosis is perhaps the most exceptional diagnostic tool that the Ayurvedic physician has at his disposal. It is based on the principle, elaborated on in this century by quantum physics, that the physical universe is essentially vibrational in nature. Every organ and tissue in the body has its own unique vibrational signature which carries the information of its state of functioning. The fluid forms of lymph and blood circulate throughout the body from heart to periphery and back again, picking up the vibrations from each organ and tissue, and conducting that vibration through *vayu*'s five different functions in the body.

Thus, the propulsive force of the heartbeat can accurately communicate a vast amount of information concerning all aspects of physiological functioning to a physician skilled in interpreting the movement or vibration in the pulse. Even the quality of mental and emotional functioning can be determined in the pulse's subtle variations.

Palpation and touch are also versatile diagnostic techniques. They can inform the physician of the functioning of all five elements by giving him knowledge of appropriate or inappropriate spaciousness, motion or vibration, temperature (inflammation or hypothermia), water content (swelling or edema) and structure (organ size and density).

Using his sense of sight, the physician can determine excess or deficient *agni* in a person's physiology through variations in coloration and complexion. Visual inspection of the patient's body, including the eyes, tongue, physiognomy, size and structure of the body, various discharges, stool and urine samples, will also give him knowledge of the state of the other four elements in the body.

Though the physician rarely, if ever, uses his sense of taste as a diagnostic tool, he frequently employs his sense of smell to determine the condition of the *bhutas*. Healthy persons usually do not exude strong odors. It is only when the tissues are at risk, as in the case of progressed cancer, that smell becomes an issue. As tissues lose the binding influence of *jala*, the structure or mass of the tissue begins to degenerate. As cellular disintegration occurs, fine particles of tissue detach and are carried out of the body in the breath, sweat, urine and feces. Odor occurs as the earth element loses its cohesion.

An Ayurvedic physician is trained to detect and discriminate among the odors that are associated with specific disease processes. For example, the ancient texts identifies twenty types of diabetes based on the specific degeneration of the tissues. Each type will discharge different cellular structures through the urine, the smell of which gives the physician a clear indication of the particular form of the disease.

The concept of *Panchamahabhuta*, the five element theory, gives us a theoretical framework for understanding *sharira*, the body. The next chapter explores the Ayurvedic understanding of the three components that make up the human physiology. It focuses on the all important theory of the three *doshas*, which is intimately associated with the theory of the five elements. The theory of *Tridosha* represents the cornerstone of Ayurvedic diagnosis and treatment. This picture of the human body that this knowledge offers is extremely rich and will demonstrate the practical value of the concepts just presented. Without it, our comprehension of the interdependent nature of the soul, mind, senses and body would be incomplete.

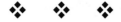

Chapter Three

DOSHA, DHATU AND *MALA:*

THE THREE COMPONENTS OF THE BODY

*M*odern medical knowledge has given us a very detailed understanding of the substances and structures that compose the human body. With the aid of modern technology, it has been able to probe deeply into the workings of organs, cells and even the minute organization of the DNA. However, even with this vast knowledge, it has not provided us with an understanding of the intelligences that initiate and coordinate all the various processes that go on within the human physiology.

What, for instance, is responsib¹ ⸱keeping certain things inside the body while separating aɪ. ⸱ɪminating other things? What determines why blood stays in and urine or feces come out? It is not enough just to say that because one is a bodily tissue, it stays in and because the other is a waste material, it is expelled.

The strength of the Ayurvedic paradigm is that it not only gives us in-depth understanding of the physical substances that compose the body but the organizing intelligences that create and govern their functions. It explains the body's composition in terms of three basic systems: *dosha, dhatu* and *mala*.

The concept of *dhatu* covers function, structure and substance, whereas the concept of *mala* is defined primarily as substance. Though both of these are included in the modern medical paradigm, Ayurveda gives them a slightly more expanded definition.

The concept of *dosha*, however, is not easily objectifiable since it cannot be understood in terms of its material substance or structure. Rather, it is more useful to understand *dosha* primarily in terms of its operational dynamics. Ayurveda derives the existence of *dosha* from extensive observation, always comparing what is happening in nature to what is going on in the body. Now, let's explore these three different components in detail to see how they work together to create *sharira*, the human body.

DHATUS: THE RETAINED SUBSTANCES AND STUCTURES OF THE BODY

Dhatu is usually translated as "body tissue," but this definition does not address some important subtleties of meaning. For most people, the term "body tissue" implies something that has structure within the body like muscle or bone. However, not all the *dhatus* appear in solid form, nor do they always have structure, as in the case of blood. They exist in many forms: liquid, semi-solid and solid.

Ayurveda, therefore, gives a definition of *dhatu* that is more precise and inclusive in its meaning. The *dhatus* are those substances and structures which are retained by the body and always rejuvenated or replenished. They are a natural part of the body's composition and give it its physical strength, structural integrity and function. In contrast to this are those substances within the body called *mala*, which are naturally expelled from the body. The concept of *mala* will be discussed shortly.

Substances are considered *dhatus* only as long as they are kept inside the body. When these "retainable" structures are expelled from the body, they are considered to be *mala* or waste matter because they no longer support the body's functioning or form part of its make-up. Injury or illness, can create situations where there is loss of blood or other fluids and tissues. If extensive enough, such unnatural loss of the *dhatus* could lead to death.

Seven *Dhatus* and their Functions

Rasa	Nutritional Fluid Plasma
Rakta	Blood - Life Force
Mamsa	Muscles - Cover Bones
Meda	Adipose Tissue - Lubrication
Asthi	Bone - Help to Stand and Walk
Majja	Bone Marrow - Nerve Tissue Nourishment
Shukra	Semen / Ovaries - Reproduction

There are seven *dhatus* which compose the retainable structures and substances of the body: *rasa* is the nutrient fluid or plasma that forms the basis of blood or *rakta*, the second *dhatu*. The third is *mamsa* or muscle tissue and the fourth is *meda* or adipose tissue (fat). *Asthi* is the term given to bone, the fifth *dhatu* and *majja* the term used to signify bone marrow and nerve tissue. The last of the seven *dhatus* is called *shukra*, the reproductive tissue of semen in the male and ovum in the female. In this text, we'll favor the Sanskrit names for the *dhatus*, since the English terms suggest meanings that are less precise.

The *dhatus* were listed in the above manner because they develop in the body in a fixed, sequential manner, one from the other. Each succeeding *dhatu* is a metabolic refinement of the previous *dhatu*, and gets nourished by it. *Rasa* (nutrient fluid) is the first *dhatu* to form, and is the metabolic end-product of the digestive processes that take place within the gastrointestinal tract. The metabolic processes that work on *rasa dhatu* then produce *rakta* (blood). Both of these *dhatus* have liquid forms and circulate all over the body.

The next *dhatus* to develop have more solid structures. *Mamsa* (muscle) comes from *rakta* (blood) and, in turn, gives rise to *meda* (fat). *Asthi* (bone) is the product of *meda* metabolism. It is the most solid of the *dhatus* and lies deep in the structure of the body. *Asthi* contains *majja*, the semi-solid substance of bone marrow and nerve tissue. *Shukra* is the last *dhatu* to be created and is the most refined. Ayurveda describes *shukra* as the semi-solid reproductive tissue which lies within the male and female reproductive systems. According to Ayurveda, *shukra* also diffuses throughout the body in subtle form. The next chapter on digestion will discuss the process of *dhatu* formation in much greater detail.

The developmental sequence of the *dhatus* is reflected in the manner in which a human fetus matures. The initial stages of fetal growth are characterized by the formation of the first *dhatus* in the series —nutrient fluid, blood and muscle tissue. The deeper *dhatus*, such as bone, marrow, and a subtle form of reproductive tissue, arise later. It takes a full nine months for all the *dhatus* to mature enough to maintain the body through their respective functions. Each works in such intimate coordination with the others that, if a baby is born prematurely, the *dhatus* will not have had time to evolve into their full functional capacities. As a result, the premature infant's ability to survive is sometimes questionable.

MALAS: THE ELIMINATED WASTES

The second component of the body as defined by Ayurveda is *mala*. The malas are those substances which the body normally discharges in the process of creating and maintaining the *dhatus*. *Mala* includes everything which is expelled because it is neither necessary for the body's support nor beneficial to it. As was mentioned previously, it also consists of any substances which are separated from the *dhatus* and eliminated when the body tries to correct imbalances. During a chest cold, for example, we expel mucus from the lungs as a by-product of the body's attempt to fight infection.

Three *Malas* and their Functions

Purisha (Feces)	Eliminates Toxins in Solid Form through Colon
Mutra (Urine)	Eliminates Toxins in Solid Form through Kidney
Sweda (Sweat)	Eliminates Toxins through Pores of Skin

Malas naturally arise as the unusable by-products of the digestive process associated with the formation of each of the seven *dhatus*. As will be explained later in the chapter, the action of the *doshas* separates this waste material from the *dhatus* at each stage of metabolism. They then get eliminated from the body in the form of fecal matter, sweat, urine, mucus, tears, saliva and carbon dioxide.

If the *malas* do not get separated from the body at the appropriate time and in the proper quantity, their accumulation causes an imbalance that damages the functioning of the *dhatus*. Everyone is familiar with the discomfort produced by constipation, a situation caused by an unhealthy retention of fecal matter in the body. If certain wastes are retained for too long, it could actually constitute a threat to life. For example, uremia is a condition that is caused by either an inability to urinate or a malfunction of the kidneys and can lead to death. Consequently, Ayurveda recommends that we never restrain any bodily urge to eliminate the *malas*.

DOSHAS: THE FUNCTIONAL INTELLIGENCES WITHIN THE BODY

The last and most significant component of the human physiology is called *dosha*. Ayurveda considers this aspect of the body to be of vital importance because it is responsible for coordinating and directing all the structures and substances of the body. Knowledge of the *doshas* and their functioning give us the understanding of the intelligence that commands the *dhatus* and *malas* and gives the body its vast functional capability. The theory of the three *doshas* is the crown jewel of Ayurvedic science and the cornerstone of all its diagnostic and treatment modalities.

The three *dosha* theory is unique to Ayurveda. With this powerful conceptual tool, the Ayurvedic physician can detect and treat patients at the earliest stages of the disease process. In fact, through the *doshic* model, a physician can locate the seeds of disease long before clear clinical symptoms appear. Countless patients visit doctors every day with vague complaints and inconclusive symptoms which indicate some deviation from balanced health. In time, these vague symptoms manifest as diseases which may be irreversible or have no effective cure. The *doshic* system, however, can make sense of these early complaints and symptoms and point to effective treatment. The Ayurvedic texts declare "that neither in theory nor in fact, is there a physical manifestation that cannot be accounted for by the concept of Tridosha." The texts show that by handling this one thing, everything gets handled.

Like the theory of *panchamahabhuta*, the three *dosha* theory has been somewhat difficult for Western medical science to grasp because it demands a more intuitive approach to studying the body. The *doshas* have no obvious material qualities like the *dhatus* or *malas*. They cannot be "objectively" studied under a microscope or in a test tube though their influence in the body is all-pervasive. As with the *mahabhutas*, Ayurveda relies on observation and comparison to understand how they work in the body.

The Relationship Between the *Bhutas* and *Doshas*

Understanding the nature of each of the five elements and their organizing principles gives us practical insight into the dynamics that drive all bodily processes. What goes on in the world at large also goes on within the human physiology. The only difference is that when the elements manifest within the body they are called *doshas*.

The question then arises, "How do the five elements become the three *doshas*?" The answer lies in the fundamental nature of each element. All five elements are responsible for orchestrating creation, yet some elements play a more active role than others. *Akash* and *prithvi*, the first and last elements to manifest, are static and unchanging in their basic nature. *Akash*, for instance, is only space and nothing exists in the emptiness of space to change. In and of itself, this element offers no resistance to change or motion, yet it provides the medium in which all change and motion occur.

Prithvi, on the other hand, has the qualities of the earth — solidity and structure-making its basic nature virtually immutable. The only time *prithvi* ever changes is under the influence of the remaining three active elements of *vayu*, *agni* and *jala*. It is in the dynamic nature of these three elements that the capacity for change and process in nature resides.

Five Elements Highlighting the Three Active Elements

Akash (Space)	Does not change
Vayu (Air) *Agni* (Fire) *Jala* (Water)	Constantly changes
Prithvi (Earth)	Does not change easily

Think about the impact of the various elements on our daily lives. We rarely give much consideration to the effects of *akash* or space on our lives unless we are on a very crowded elevator, and we tend to take for granted the relative stability of earth unless we are in an earthquake. We do, however, pay a great deal of attention to *vayu* (air or wind), *agni* (heat) and *jala* (water), because of the tremendous influence they have on everyday life. We are constantly measuring and monitoring them. Every time we look out the window, we take into account the condition of these three *bhutas*. Meteorologists and other scientists regularly study wind and storm patterns, earthquakes, temperature changes, rainfall and relative humidity.

Vayu, which is commonly associated with the wind, is responsible for all motion as well as all drying functions in nature. When *vayu* is balanced, it operates like a benevolent director of transportation, causing everything in creation to move in a smooth, orderly fashion so that it arrives in the right place at the right time.

Because *vayu* controls all movement in nature, it actually governs the actions of the other two dynamic elements. For example, a rain cloud contains both *jala*, in the form of moisture, and *agni*, in the form of lightning. However, without *vayu*'s impulse for movement, the cloud cannot move and it cannot release its water or lightning. *Vayu*, in fact, governs all weather patterns and natural events. When *vayu* goes out of balance, it drives the wind into cyclones and hurricanes and is responsible for volcanic eruptions. *Vayu* can whip the ocean into huge waves, and shake the earth.

Agni, the fire element, manifests the properties of heat and light and facilitates all transformations. It is associated with the sun, whose energies are essential to life, and regulates temperature, keeping it within the narrow range necessary to maintain life. Without light and heat, none of the metabolic activities which convert nutrients into energy and structure would be possible. *Agni*'s balanced functioning plays a critical role in the life of the planet. With too little heat, all conversion processes would come to a halt. With too much heat, all processes would accelerate until everything was completely consumed.

Fluidity and cohesion characterize *jala*, the water element. Associated with the moon, *jala* influences the ocean tides and the ebb and flow of fluids in the body. Due to *jala*'s binding quality, when humidity rises, things stick together. *Jala* manifests as rainfall, and when it is balanced, rain comes on time and in sufficient quantity to provide cohesion and nourishment to the earth. Growth results largely from *jala*'s nature to add, unit by unit.

Just as these active elements control all processes in creation, so also do the three *doshas* perform similar functions within the body, regulating all movement, transformation and liquefaction. The *doshas* are the *bhutas* in microform. As such, they take on the qualities associated with their respective *bhutas*.

Elements which Become *Dosha's* in the Body

Akash (Space) *Vayu* (Air)	*Vata Dosha*
Agni (Fire)	*Pitta Dosha*
Jala (Water) *Prithvi* (Earth)	*Kapha Dosha*

It would be incorrect to think of the *doshas* only as the three dynamic elements manifesting in the body. These active elements are always supported by the two unchanging elements, for change can only happen upon the foundation of non-change. Thus, *vayu* and *akash* combine to become *vata dosha*, which controls all aspects of movement as well as space within the body. In spite of this combination, however, *vata dosha* tends to primarily display the characteristics of *vayu* — the wind. The words," dry, light, cold, quick, rough, minute" and "mobile" describe the characteristics of *vata dosha*.

Agni, in conjunction with some of the qualities of *vayu* and *jala*, becomes *pitta dosha*. This is the function that governs all the body's conversion processes as well as its heat and energy producing capacities. *Pitta dosha* is primarily characterized by the qualities of *agni*, which are hot, sharp, penetrating, light, acidic and slightly oily.

Jala supported by *prithvi*, becomes *kapha dosha* and controls liquefaction, lubrication and cohesion. It is also responsible for giving solidity and structure to the body. *Kapha dosha* primarily reflects the qualities of water, but also has some traits of the earth element. Consequently, *kapha* is heavy, slow, cold, steady, solid and oily.

Another interesting feature of the *doshas* is that each has a taste associated with it. *Vata* is mostly pungent; *pitta* is sour and *kapha* is sweet. The utility of this knowledge will become more apparent in the next chapter. Now, let's continue with our explanation of the *dosha*'s pervasive influence in the body.

The *Doshas'* Zones in the Body

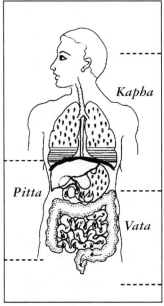

The three zones of the body

Each *bhuta* or element dominates the quality of life in specific geographical areas of the world. Some places are dry, reflecting the qualities of *vayu*; some are hot, indicating that *agni* is in greater abundance there; while others are very moist or humid, demonstrating the predominance of *jala*. Is it possible that this same phenomenon is reflected in the way the *doshas* function in our body? Does each *dosha* exert a dominant influence in a particular zone or "geographical" location in the human body?

To determine this, it is helpful to think of the G-I tract as a long, hollow tube extending from the mouth to the anus. This tube and the area of the body surrounding it can be divided into three segments according to the specific function that each seems to have in the body.

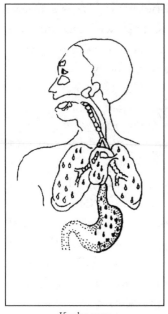

Kapha zone

Kapha Zone

Let's first examine the upper part of the body from the head to the diaphragm. The organs in this area include the sense organs, tongue, larynx, pharynx, esophagus, trachea, lungs, bronchi, heart, pericardium and upper part of the stomach. Notice that these organs produce moisture in the form of watery secretions which are essential to the body. For instance, the tongue produces saliva which mixes with food and liquefies it enough to be swallowed. The eyes and nose secrete moisture to protect themselves and maintain their function. Membranes in the lungs secrete mucus to prevent them from drying out. The functions of these organs are associated with the qualities of *kapha* — moistening, mixing, binding together and lubricating — the same activities performed in nature by *jala*. Other parts of the body produce secretions, but they have a different purpose.

This zone is not only characterized by more secretions (*jala*), but also by more structure (*prithvi*) than in any other part of the body. Witness the cranium, the jaw and facial structure, the shoulders, clavicle and rib cage. The large amount of structure in this part of the body is another indication of the predominant influence of *kapha* manifesting through *prithvi* or the earth element. Because of the structure and function of this section of the body, Ayurveda calls it the *kapha* zone.

Secretions or discharges in this part of the body, like saliva or mucus, tend to be mainly white or pale because of their *kaphic* or watery nature. Foods which increase the water and earth elements in the body, like milk and bananas, also show this whitish color. Most grains reflect a predominantly *kaphic* quality as well. When

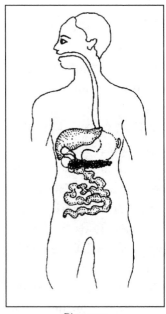

Pitta zone

ground into flour, all grains are white and their taste is sweet; they tend to be heavy and increase body weight. *Kaphic* foods nourish the body and add substance to it.

Pitta Zone

Now let's look at the next section of the body from the diaphragm to the umbilicus. This zone covers the lower part of the stomach, the small intestine up to the ileocecal valve, the liver, pancreas, gallbladder and spleen. Each of these organs produces substances containing acids or enzymes which are responsible for chemical transformation. These include hydrochloric acid, digestive enzymes, pancreatic juices and bile.

Clearly, the primary purpose of this part of the body is conversion, the function of *pitta dosha* in the body. The secretions in this zone change the structure, color and quality of whatever they contact.

Whereas the lubricating and cohesive secretions of the *kapha* zone appear dull whitish, sticky and opaque, the *pitta* zone produces substances in a variety of colors, especially yellow, red and green. Just as *agni*, in the form of sunlight, contains all the hues of the rainbow, so *agni* manifesting in the body as *pitta* secretions also come in many shades. Foods such as spices have high levels of *agni* and come in an array of bright colors. These heat-producing *pitta* foods stimulate the conversion process in the body. We eat them in much smaller amounts than *kaphic* foods, because they would have too heating an influence on the body if eaten in larger quantities.

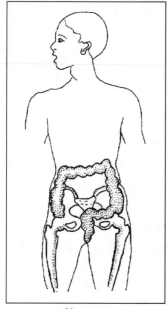

Vata zone

Vata Zone

The last section of the body to examine extends from the navel downwards and includes the large intestine, the reproductive organs, the organs of elimination and the legs. Porosity, space, dryness, lightness and movement describe the functions of this region. The organs here do not produce secretions, but rather re-absorb fluids back into the body or hold fluids to be excreted from it. Both the organs and the bones in this region are larger and have more space inside them than those in the other two zones of the body. This is due to the predominance of *akash* and *vayu*, the two elements that constitute *vata dosha* in the body. For example, compared to the small intestine in the *pitta* zone, the colon in the *vata* zone has a larger diameter, greater porosity and dryness, and a darker color.

Vata controls the mechanisms involved in drying and separating food. As *vata* moves food residue through the large intestine, the substance becomes dehydrated, it darkens and is finally expelled from the body. We find dark colors here, such as brown, purple or black. Though the colon is the primary seat of *vata* in the body, the bones are also home to *vata*. This is seen especially in the composition of the pelvic bones, which are large, porous and hard with the strength to support the majority of the body's weight.

There are food substances that can be identified as *vata*-promoting foods based on their inherent qualities. These foods, such as staple foods (legumes, beans etc.), are hard, rough and dry and have a darker color. Foods which easily give up their water, like watermelon, are also *vata* foods.

Each of these areas or zones of the body has a specific function intimately linked to the properties of each *dosha*. The reigning *dosha* plays a highly significant role in the health of each physiological zone, because of its specialized ability to remove imbalances in the organs and tissues of that zone.

Though *kapha*, *pitta*, and *vata* each have their separate domains, they are also found pervading the entire body. *Vata*, however, has the most universal influence. It governs the ability to respond to stimuli and is responsible for moving *kapha* and *pitta* throughout the body. For example, when we are thirsty, *vata* moves us to get water, brings the glass to our mouth, allows us to swallow, carries the water through our digestive tract and to the tissues. With *vata*'s help, the secretions of the *kapha* and *pitta* zones flow from their source to where they are needed. Oxygen, nourishment, waste products and toxins are all moved by *vata*.

Vata animates life; it initiates and maintains all of life's essential processes. Everything we do consumes energy and, from the moment of birth, all energy expenditure is orchestrated by *vata*. When a baby is born, the first thing it does is to cry. This act of crying uses the energy that was stored in the baby's *dhatus*. This energy must be expended before the baby can draw in air to begin breathing on its own.

The *Doshas* and the Stages of Life

How pervasive is the influence of the three *doshas* in human life? Not only do they govern specific areas of the body and their functioning, they regulate the physical and psychological development of various stages of life. Just as we divided the body into three distinct segments according to the dominant influence of a particular *dosha*, so we can divide our life span.

Kapha Stage

Look, for instance, at the initial stage of human development, from birth through puberty. This phase is characterized by nourishment and growth in the body's substance and size. This phase is called the *kapha* age because one of the main qualities of this *dosha* is that it adds, unit by unit. It is because of this quality that children continue to grow and accumulate body mass regardless of what or whether they eat. They naturally have a greater amount of fatty tissue, which is also characteristic of *kapha*. During these early years, *kapha*-related disorders, such as colds, sinus, allergies, ear and respiratory infections, are the most common ailments. Notice that these illnesses all occur within the *kapha* zone of the body.

Pitta Stage

In the next stage of life, which begins at puberty, we notice that the body's growth potential is suddenly converted into reproductive potential and the increase in mass and size begins to slow down. The body develops distinct sexual characteristics and *shukra dhatu* becomes active, creating semen in the male and ovum in the female.

The transforming quality of this stage continues to manifest well into middle age, but after puberty, it takes on a more psychological nature. During these *pitta* years, the increased "fire" gives people ambition, courage, energy and motivation to achieve their goals and overcome obstacles. We see mainly *pitta*-related disorders arising during this time, including skin disorders, food allergies, hyperacidity and other digestive disturbances.

Vata Stage

Around middle age, we notice something new starting to happen to the mind and body. Our drive starts to wane. The skin begins to dry and wrinkle. The body becomes more frail and may lose weight, and the muscles start to lose some of their tone and flexibility. Hair thins and grays. Strength and stamina gradually decrease and the mind loses its clarity. The system is starting to feel the drying, separating and immobilizing effects of *vata dosha* as it dominates this phase of human life. *Vata*'s influence brings a natural tendency toward dehydration: tissues waste away and the natural cycles of metabolic activity are disrupted.

The diseases which most frequently appear at this time are *vata*-related disorders, such as insomnia, sensory depletion (loss of hearing and weakened eye sight), memory loss, anxiety and various degenerative and neurological problems. To prevent *doshic* imbalances and disease, this stage demands that we pay much more attention to diet and lifestyle than we did during the first two stages of life.

All living things, without exception, grow, reproduce and die in this natural *kapha-pitta-vata* cycle. We see the same cycle occurring in the plant and animal kingdoms as we see in human life. For instance, as a seed sprouts and grows into a seedling, it absorbs more and more water and nutrients and rapidly increases in size. It is green, soft, and tender. When the plant matures, it stops growing in size; it hardens and its color darkens. It produces flowers, fruits and seeds. In the last phase of its life, the plant becomes dehydrated and shrinks. No matter how much water and fertilizer it gets, it continues to shrivel until it dies.

During the *kapha* and *pitta* stages of life, disease symptoms may sometimes be suppressed. However, once *vata*'s influence takes over, the body can no longer hide nor mask symptoms, and occasional discomforts turn into debilitating disorders. *Vata*'s mobile potency easily concentrates toxins in weak *dhatus*, where they disrupt the *dhatus*' metabolism and deprive them of nutrition. *Vata*'s drying tendency dehydrates the *dhatus* and impairs immunity. Toxins and wastes may accumulate in the body during the *kapha* and *pitta* periods, but the evidence of degenerative disease will usually start to appear with the onset of the *vata* stage of life. This is when individuals becomes aware that they have serious health problems. Diseases which could have been easily prevented in earlier years now become difficult to treat because their manifestation is supported by an irreversible cycle of nature.

The *Doshas* and the Seasons

The degree of influence that each element demonstrates in nature varies with geographical location, the seasons, the climate and the time of day. *Vayu* produces motion, drying and the separation of particles. Its influence can be seen dominating in the late afternoon; in the autumn, when dry winds blow; in deserts and on windy mountains. *Agni* brings heat and transformation. It rules at midday, when the sun is at its apex; during the summer; and in tropical environments, where things grow and decay rapidly. *Jala*, which provides moisture, fluidity and cohesion, is strong early in the morning, when dew settles on the leaves of plants; in the springtime, when rain moistens the earth and nourishes plant life; and in damp, cool forests.

Kapha Season

The dominance of a particular element in the environment heightens or minimizes each *dosha*'s effect on its respective physiological zone, as well as on the body in general. External conditions strongly impact internal conditions. When *jala* dominates the environment, *kapha*'s physiological action intensifies. As water increases in the atmosphere in the form of rain or snow, most people will tend to experience increased watery secretions in the body. Too much of this watery influence can cause *kapha dosha* to become excessive or imbalanced. When cold, wetness and heaviness get strong enough to overwhelm and diminish *pitta*'s heat, we develop colds, head or chest congestion, sinusitis, watery eyes, etc. Common sense gives us the key to maintaining good health in cold conditions: counterbalance powerful environmental conditions by managing the body, i.e. dress warmly and take warm food and beverages.

Pitta Season

When *agni*'s influence pervades the environment, *pitta*'s influence on the body intensifies. The hot climates in jungles and deserts, as well as summer's high temperatures, indicate *agni*'s dominance. If *pitta* is not controlled to counteract increased heat in the environment, the body's conversion processes accelerate, causing both internal and external burning or inflammation, as well as an increase in heated emotions, like anger and irritability. *Pitta* in the physiology will spontaneously decrease when the *agni* in the environment does, in cooler seasons and climates.

Vata Season

Vata takes control in the autumn, when the weather turns cool, windy and often dry. *Vata* can easily become excessive at this time, when it dominates the liquefying function of *kapha* and the heating function of *pitta*. Since *vata* governs motion and produces dehydration, it can cause dryness in the moving parts of the body, such as joints and muscles, and can create the stiffness and aches associated with the flu. If *vata* is not kept balanced during this season, it can cause other health problems associated with dryness and mobility, such as constipation, dry skin, coldness, anxiety and insomnia. *Vata* also has a dominant influence in the spring.

The *Doshas* and the Time of Day

In addition to the effect that the active elements have on the seasons and geographical areas, they also dominate particular times of day. One element will exert a stronger influence over the others during a particular four-hour period. This elemental cycle of influence is actually repeated twice in every twenty-four-hour period, beginning at sunrise. From six to ten in the morning, when the air is heavy, cold, and damp with dew, *jala* is strongest. Later in the morning, the sun begins to exert its power, burning away the cold and damp. *Agni* then dominates the day between ten and two, when the sun is at its height. After two o'clock, *vayu* takes over, producing its cool, dry and windy influence. Anyone who has lived by the ocean understands these cycles. The sea is calm in the morning, but by late in the day it becomes rough, whipped by the afternoon winds.

This cycle is duplicated in the following twelve-hour period. After sunset, *jala* again gains ascendancy, generating more dampness, heaviness and cold in the atmosphere. During the two hours before and after midnight — *agni*'s time — the weather steadies and the light of the stars appear brighter. From two in the morning until sunrise, when *vayu* is predominating, the air becomes a little dryer and more active.

The daily flow of the elements effects our bodies through the *doshas*. Around sunrise, the water element elevates, causing more *kapha* secretions to flow from the *dhatus* into the G-I tract. At midday, *agni*'s time, *pitta* secretions in the G-I tract increase, causing hunger and thirst, and the body's conversion processes function at maximum strength. In the late afternoon and early morning, before dawn, when *vayu* is at its height, the body experiences more movement, and eliminative processes are most active.

During their respective periods of dominance, an excess accumulation of each *dosha* forms in the dense, solid *dhatus*. Gravity exerts its force on these accumulations, and they naturally drain into the lighter, more hollow structures of the body. The *doshas* travel from the *dhatus* to the internal mucous membranes, where they become more available in the G-I tract. This twice-daily movement of the *doshas* plays an important role in Ayurvedic medicine. Later chapters discuss in detail how the rejuvenative science of *Panchakarma* takes advantage of this flow to eliminate *dosha*-specific impurities from the physiology.

The Role of the *Doshas*

Now that we understand the relationship between the *doshas* and the elements, we can examine the *doshas* in terms of their functions in the body, especially the effects they have on the *dhatus* and *malas*. The Ayurvedic texts define *dosha* as that which is neither retained nor eliminated by the body. The *doshas* do not exist as retainable structures or materials, like the *dhatus*, nor are they substances which the body eliminates, like the *malas*. They have little or no obvious material form, and they cannot be easily seen or examined directly. The *doshas* play an active but somewhat invisible role in orchestrating the processes that create and sustain the body.

Dhatu and *mala* cannot operate by themselves. *Dhatu* lacks the ability to nourish itself, and *mala* cannot eliminate itself from the body. They depend on the intelligence of the *doshas* to direct them. When in balance, the *doshas* know exactly when and where to go in the body and how to manage the processes of nourishment and elimination. Their ability to coordinate and administrate the function of the *dhatus* and *malas* makes them extremely important in Ayurveda.

Doshas and Their Function

Vata Dosha	Separation / Movement
Pitta Dosha	Conversion / Transformation
Kapha Dosha	Cohesion / Liquidity

It is useful to think of the *doshas* as agents of change. They make things happen. They are the unseen forces that do all the transporting, transforming and packaging in the body. *Vata* acts as a vehicle which carries nutrients from one stage of the digestive process to the next. It collects waste products from each stage of metabolism and returns them to the gastrointestinal tract for elimination. *Pitta* transforms the food substances brought to it by *vata* into more nourishing products, which *vata* then distributes to the *dhatus*. *Kapha* serves as a medium of transport, binding together food stuffs ready to be transformed, nutrients ready to be distributed and waste products ready to be expelled.

Dosha's uniqueness as a functional intelligence is demonstrated in a remarkable ability that is not possessed by either *dhatu* or *mala*. Ayurveda describes this special capacity as *dosha gati*, the movement of the *doshas* back and forth between the body's more solid structures and its hollow structures. This is a very crucial ability. Unlike the *malas*, the *doshas* can move from the gastrointestinal tract to the *dhatus*. The three *doshas* act together as a carrier vehicle, whose function is to bring food, oxygen and water from the internal mucous membranes of the G-I tract to the superficial and deep tissues constituting the *dhatus*.

Unlike the *dhatus*, the *doshas* can move from the *dhatus* to the gastrointestinal tract. Again, they act in unison to transport metabolic by-products and toxins from the *dhatus* to the internal mucous membranes for elimination. *Dosha* functions between *dhatu* and *mala*, influencing their condition and status in the body. It combines with *dhatu* and *mala* without itself being changed or harmed.

We see this concept at work in our salivary glands. When we are hungry and someone puts a delicious meal in front of us, we suddenly begin to salivate. The food we eat mixes with the saliva in our mouths so that it becomes liquid enough to be swallowed. How did the saliva appear? The *doshas* brought it from the solid and semi-solid *dhatus* to the hollow structure of the mouth. Once they have done their job, these secretions will be reabsorbed from the stomach and intestines and carried back to the *dhatus* by the action of the *doshas*.

Dosha gati is also instrumental in helping the *doshas* maintain water balance in the body. Urination is more frequent when we are relaxing than when we are exerting ourselves. During periods of low activity, the *dhatus* or tissues do not need as much fluid to lubricate and protect them. The *doshas* keep the balance of tissue-fluid by removing excess water from the *dhatus* to the body's hollow structures. When we become more active, we develop a thirst, the body's signal that the *dhatus* need moisture. The *doshas* carry the fluid we drink to the specific *dhatus* that are in need.

When an Ayurvedic physician understands where the dysfunction is occurring in the digestive process, he can determine which *dosha* is aggravated or blocked. Thus, proper use of the appropriate *ahara* (diet) and *vihara* (exercise) methods to eliminate the imbalance can be applied.

If we study *vihar* treatments, as explained in Ayurveda, *yogasanas* and *pranayama* are recommended to balance the *doshas*.

If we observe *asanas*, we can see clearly that they regulate the *doshas*.

In observing a specific *asana* (posture), such as one specifically designed to work on the abdomen, we see that it increases pressure on the organs, which in turn assists those organs (*dhatus*) to release *ama*. When the posture is released, expansion follows, which increases the nutrition and oxygenation to all the organs in the abdominal cavity. This enhances the elimination of the *malas* from the body, which promotes nutrition and helps to increase *agni* for stronger metabolism.

So, *yogasanas* have been designed in Ayurveda to enhance the ability of *doshas* to maintain proper *dhatu* and *mala* functions. I would suggest that the sages in India created *yogasana* mainly to regulate the *doshas* in the body. I will discuss more about this in *Vihara chikitsa*, (pages 146-151).

The following four premises describe *doshic* functioning. Their importance for healing and rejuvenating the body is paramount and will be elaborated on in detail in the second section of this book.

(i) The *doshas* can move anywhere in the body, from the deepest structures of bone marrow and reproductive tissue to the surface of the skin and back again.

(ii) The *doshas'* intelligence discriminates between what the body should retain and what it should eliminate, and acts accordingly.

(iii) Each *dosha* is most efficient in eliminating impurities that accumulate in its own zone of functioning as well as promoting nutrition in that particular zone.

(iv) The *dosha*'s twice-daily migration periods are the best times for the movement of waste products from the body's

deeper structures to its hollow structures and the movement of nutritional products from the G-I tract to the
deep tissues.

The next chapter will discuss the intimate connection between
doshic function, digestion and health. When an Ayurvedic physician understands where dysfunction is occurring in the digestive
process, he can determine which *dosha* is "aggravated" and use the
appropriate methods to eliminate the imbalance.

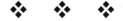

Chapter Four

DIGESTION: THE KEY TO HEALTH

*W*ith the knowledge contained in the last three chapters, we now have a solid foundation for understanding the actual processes that create and sustain the body. Digestion plays a very key role in Ayurveda's understanding of human health and illness. Though Ayurveda contends that all diseases originate first in the mind, on a physical level this invariably manifests as a breakdown in metabolic function. Because of this, it gives great importance to the process of digestion, whereas modern medicine places much less emphasis on the body's metabolic processes as the source of either health or disease.

Ayurvedic science offers an elaborate and detailed description of the body's metabolic functions and their relationship to organ and tissue formation. It confirms the importance of efficient food conversion to supply the nutrients which enable each *dhatu* to perform its job. It also recognizes that health requires the proper elimination of the natural by-products occurring from the digestive processes.

A rough analogy can be drawn to a car engine. When fuel combustion in the cylinders is inefficient, the compression lowers and the car responds sluggishly. In addition, carbon produced by incomplete combustion starts to form deposits on valves and other parts of the engine, further damaging the engine's compression and interfering with the car's performance. In a similar manner, if metabolic conversion of food is incomplete, it can produce sluggishness or low energy. The undigested food material also becomes the source for degenerative diseases.

The *Doshas* and Digestion

In the previous chapter we briefly explained that the *dhatus* are formed sequentially, one being a metabolic refinement of the previous one. Proper formation of the *dhatus* requires the complete and efficient breakdown of nutrients supplied to the metabolic staging ground of that *dhatu* from the previous stages. It is therefore vital for health that metabolism be strong in all seven stages.

What then is responsible for strong, efficient digestion? As was mentioned in the previous chapter, neither the *dhatus* nor the *malas* have the specific ability to accomplish these complex metabolic functions. Only *vayu*, *agni* and *jala*, acting as *vata*, *pitta* and *kapha doshas* in the body, possess the specific intelligence sufficient to conduct these processes. Ultimately, everything to do with metabolic function and its relationship to health and disease boils down to the coordinated actions of the three *doshas*.

The disease process starts when the *doshas'* natural relationship becomes imbalanced or impaired. *Doshic* action and digestion are locked in a functional interdependence in which an impairment in one necessarily involves an impairment in the other. When one or more of the *doshas* becomes deficient or excessive in their functioning, indigestion results.

Each *dosha* displays a twice-daily cycle of predominance, reflecting the influence of its respective *bhuta* in the environment. However, when a *dosha's* dominance continues outside the normal time period, it becomes "aggravated." An aggravated *dosha* no longer interacts in a balanced manner with the other two. It overwhelms them and inhibits their ability to perform their respective operations. Whether it's *kapha's* ability to liquefy and bind, *pitta's* capacity to transform, or *vata's* ability to separate and transport, their activity becomes weak or sluggish,. The precise coordination of all three of these functions is critical to healthy digestion.

The *doshas* perform many functions within the body, but in

regards to the processes concerned with transforming foodstuffs into nutrients for the *dhatus*, *pitta dosha* has the most crucial role. The question then arises as to the relationship between *agni*, the vital force in the body and *pitta dosha*.

Relationship Between *Agni* and *Pitta*

A key concept in the Ayurvedic understanding of digestion is "digestive fire," the process responsible for metabolic conversion within the body. Anything having to do with heat, light, conversion or transformation anywhere in the universe is under the control of the *bhuta* or element of *agni*. In the body, however, *agni* turns over some of its functions to *pitta dosha*. Before we proceed further with our discussion of digestion, it will be useful to clarify the roles that *agni* and *pitta dosha* have in the body.

Agni's role in human physiology covers a multitude of functions. It produces vigor and vitality, the glow of the complexion, sight, thermogenesis and the structure of the *dhatus*. In fact, *agni* is responsible for life itself. In the context of the digestive processes that occur in the G-I tract, *agni bhuta* is called *jathara agni*.

Jathara agni manifests more specifically in the body as the five forms or sub-*doshas* of *pitta*. Each of these has a specific metabolic function and location in the body. The most important of these sub-*doshas* for our discussion here is *pachak pitta*, which is found in the lower stomach and small intestine, and is referred to by Ayurveda as the "digestive fire." This function of *pitta* is what is responsible for our appetite and digestive ability.

Five Types of *Pitta* and their Locations

Pachak Pitta	Small Intestine
Ranjak Pitta	Liver
Alochak Pitta	Eyes
Sadhak Pitta	Brain
Bhrajak Pitta	Skin

The other four digestive activities of *pitta* which are closely related to *pachak pitta*'s activities are *ranjak*, which controls the liver function; *alochak*, found in the eye and is responsible for digesting visual images; *bhrajak*, located in the skin and is responsible for complexion; and finally *sadhak pitta*, which controls thought metabolism.

Just as *agni bhuta* manifests in the G-I tract in the form of *jathara agni* or *pachak pitta*, it also appears as the metabolic function responsible for creating and maintaining all seven *dhatus*. In this role, *agni* is known as the seven *dhatu agnis*.

Though *jathara agni* and the *dhatu agnis* have their respective *pitta* functions, it is important to understand the distinction between *agni* and *pitta*. As an element, *agni* has no distinguishable form in the body; it cannot be identified by material qualities. However, when it appears as *pitta dosha*, it is perceptible, because it becomes cloaked in the characteristics of all five elements. For instance, when *jathara agni* appears as *pachak pitta*, it exhibits properties that are characteristic of digestive enzymes and acid secretions, i.e., it has a slightly oily, liquid quality that moves or flows. It also has a distinctly sour odor and taste, and a yellow, green or reddish color.

Another important difference is that *agni*'s basic nature is to convert and consume, a process that never stops. When no food is available to convert, *agni* digests the oily and liquid substances of *pitta* and *kapha doshas*. When that is gone, it starts to consume the *dhatus*. This explains why fasting or starvation produces emaciation. In contrast, when there is no longer food to digest, *pitta* leaves the gastrointestinal tract and is eliminated as *mala*, the bile which gives the feces its brown color.

When both the digestive fire or *pachak pitta* are strong and in balance, the appetite is good without being excessive and digestion goes on almost unnoticed. Moderate eating satisfies us. We feel light and energized after eating and do not experience any strong food cravings. Food gets completely metabolized and the refined end-products of digestion move to the right tissues, in the right quantity to nourish the *dhatus*. Since proper metabolism is so crucial to health, it is important to first understand what causes digestion to malfunction and why Ayurveda links it to the formation of almost all disease processes.

Indigestion and *Ama*

Most people would define indigestion as the temporary inconvenience or discomfort that arises from eating too much food or eating foods that are too rich or spicy for our digestive process to handle. This description tends to place the focus more on the symptoms of indigestion than the process itself. Ayurveda offers a much more specific and comprehensive definition. It states that indigestion is both the inability to transform and assimilate food and the inability to eliminate metabolic waste products that result from the digestive process. Several things occur as a result of poor digestion.

First, *ama* forms in the G-I tract. *Ama* is the food which remains in the gastrointestinal tract in undigested form. It is different from *mala*, which, as we defined earlier, is the natural, unusable waste-product resulting from healthy metabolism. If the toxic sticky residue of incomplete metabolism (*ama*) is not quickly burned up by the digestive fire, it will accumulate in the G-I tract.

When *ama* becomes too plentiful in this area, it will naturally be removed by the *doshas* and transported to the *dhatus* by the action of *dosha gati* — the twice-daily movement of the *doshas* from the G-I tract to the deeper tissues of the body. Once *ama* is deposited in the *dhatus*, it begins a chain of events that debilitates them and impairs their function. This results in a weakened immune system that makes the *dhatus* susceptible to infection and degenerative disease.

Second, *ama* interferes with or "spoils" the functioning of the *doshas*, leading to a breakdown in their coordination. This dysfunction especially disturbs or depletes the strength of the digestive *agni*, in the form of *pachak pitta*, which becomes responsible for the creation of even more *ama* — undigested food stuff.

Third, when digestion is impaired, nutritional products are not available to nourish the *dhatus*. Metabolism and assimilation of nutrients for *dhatu* development happens sequentially. When the refinement process breaks down in one stage, all succeeding stages are adversely affected.

Fourth, the natural *doshic* processes that eliminate *mala* get disturbed. As a result of an imbalance in *vata* functioning caused by *ama*, metabolic waste products can no longer be properly removed from the *dhatus* and carried back to the G-I tract for elimination. This accumulation of waste further weakens and damages the *dhatus*.

Lastly, the *ama* and *mala* which have accumulated block the *dhatus* ability to assimilate food and medicine, so it becomes difficult for them to regain their healthy status. *Ama* can remain in the *dhatus* for years, and tends to accumulate in those *dhatus* which are congenitally weak or have been most damaged by *ama*'s influence in the past.

All these factors contribute to the *dhatus*' impaired functioning and constitute the root cause of most degenerative diseases. The extensive diagnostic techniques available to an Ayurvedic physician allow him to locate in which *dhatus* the *ama* has been deposited, and the extent of the dysfunction and physical damage. Diagnosis also pinpoints the imbalances in the digestive process which were responsible for producing the *ama* in the first place. We will discuss this later in the chapter, after we have elaborated on the Ayurvedic understanding of the two phases of digestion.

TWO PHASES OF DIGESTION

Ayurveda explains that digestion occurs not only in the gastrointestinal tract but in the *dhatus* as well, and makes a clear distinction between these two different metabolic processes. The conversion that takes place in the gastrointestinal tract, up to and including absorption through the intestinal walls, is called *prapaka* digestion. This initial stage of digestion prepares the food we eat to be assimilated by the *dhatus* in the next seven metabolic stages, known collectively as *vipaka* digestion, the post-absorptive digestive processes.

PRAPAKA METABOLISM: DIGESTION IN THE G-I TRACT

Recall in our discussion of the *doshas* that the gastrointestinal tract and the area surrounding it is divided into three sections according to the *dosha*-specific functions which govern that area. The upper part of the G-I tract is dominated by the cohesive, liquefying and lubricating functions of *kapha dosha*; the middle zone by the transformative actions of *pitta dosha* and the lower section by the drying, separating and absorptive processes of *vata dosha*.

Each of these zones actively participates in the first or *prapaka* stage of digestion.

Prapaka digestion begins with eating and swallowing. As the food moves through the G-I tract, *jathara agni* causes it to undergo a fixed sequence of metabolic actions which are determined by the *dosha*-specific functions of the zone in which they are occurring. These three stages of *prapaka* digestion are referred to as the three transient phases of metabolism.

Three Phases of *Prapak* (Transient) Metabolism

Prapak Metabolism	Dosha Zone	Taste	Function
Madhur	*Kapha*	Sweet	Moistening of food
Amla	*Pitta*	Sour	Conversion of food
Katu	*Vata*	Pungent	Absorption and Separation of food

Another important point to remember from Chapter Three is that each *dosha* has associated with it a dominant taste or *rasa*. The inherent natures of the five elements and their combinations give rise to six basic tastes: sweet, sour, salty, bitter, pungent and astringent. However, when the elements specifically combine to form the *doshas* in the body, they give rise to a taste characteristically associated with that particular *dosha*.

When the water and earth elements combine to form *kapha dosha*, a sweet taste is always created. Keep in mind that when Ayurveda refers to the sweet taste associated with *kapha*, they are not talking about the highly concentrated sweetness found in foods made with refined sugars. The taste inherent to the nature of *agni bhuta* is sour, which makes the taste associated with *pitta dosha* predominantly sour. When *akash* and *vayu* combine to form *vata dosha*, they form a primarily pungent taste.

What is the significance of taste to *prapaka* digestion? As food moves through the three *dosha*-specific stages of *prapaka*, or transient digestion, it takes on the taste associated with the *dosha* governing that particular zone. The influence of *jathara agni* will first cause the whole food mass to be converted to a predominantly sweet taste in the *kapha* zone, then to a sour taste in the *pitta* zone and finally to a pungent taste in the *vata* zone. These basic tastes will predominate regardless of the taste the food has at the time it was eaten.

When we eat food, it first enters the *kapha* zone, the first stage of transient metabolism, where it gets moistened and liquefied. Because of the abundance of watery secretions in this zone, the food also increases in volume. Even if the food mass contains all six tastes, it acquires a predominantly sweet taste, and foods that already have a sweet flavor will become even sweeter in this initial phase of *prapaka* digestion.

As the food moves into the second phase of transient digestion in the mid-zone, *agni*'s qualities begin to take over. Temperature rises due to the conversion process taking place. The particles of food which were bound together and liquefied by *kapha*'s action now mix with acid secretions from glands in the *pitta* zone. They are broken down and homogenized and can no longer be recognized as distinct particles of food. As a whole, the food mass takes on the sour taste associated with *pitta dosha*.

During the final stage of transient metabolism, the transformed food mass enters *vata* territory, where absorption begins. Under *vata*'s influence, the food's nutrient portions are separated from the parts that can't be used. In this process, *jala* (water) gets separated from *prithvi* (earth) and, as a consequence, the food mass decreases in volume. Though *jathara agni* is still active in this last phase of *prapaka* digestion, the food mass becomes largely pungent in taste, a quality of *vata* that is due to the absence of the water element.

The Universal Nature of Transient Metabolism

This metabolic sequence is not unique to human physiology; it is a universal phenomenon. *Jathara agni* exerts its influence on life everywhere, particularly organic life, and we see the same three transient phases operating throughout nature. For example, freshly cooked rice is sweeter than uncooked rice, reflecting the sweet phase of transient metabolism. If this rice is left outside, the *agni* in the environment soon causes it to become acidic and turn sour. Because of this transformation, it becomes more homogenous and less recognizable as individual rice particles. Having passed through the transient sweet and sour phases, the rice enters the pungent phase. It begins to bubble, as the water in the rice separates from the solid particles. Here again we see *vata*'s influence causing *jala* to separate from *prithvi*.

The progressive influence of *jathara agni* can again be seen when milk or fruit is left unrefrigerated in warm weather. At first, the milk and fruit are sweet and the *prithvi* and *jala* in their makeup are well contained. After a time, the fruit and milk begin to taste sour or acidic. Finally, they decompose and the water and solids separate. The fruit becomes mealy and dry, and the milk curdles. Both substances take on a pungent smell.

If we were to eat a few slices of fresh bread, a sweet food, and then regurgitate a small amount after a few minutes, we would find the bread had become even sweeter and more liquid than it was originally. If we regurgitated some of the bread a few hours later, after it has entered the small intestine, we would find it had a sour taste and a homogenous appearance which is unrecognizable as bread. If, after more time, the food mass could be examined in the colon, or its by-product examined in the excrement, it would be drier in appearance and have a pungent smell. This demonstrates the progressive influence of *jathara agni* in *prapaka* digestion.

The Influence of the Three Transient Phases on the Body

As food moves through the three transient phases of *prapaka* digestion, the whole body feels the influence of each *dosha* as it sequentially dominates digestion. In the first stage, the influence of *kapha* creates a heavy, or even a sleepy feeling. When food leaves the stomach and enters *pitta*'s zone, conversion processes elevate body temperature and we begin to feel warm and thirsty. When our food enters the last phase, the influence of *vata* stimulates in us the need for activity.

We can see these three transient phases affecting animals in much the same way. If you have a dog, notice that soon after the dog has eaten it will become lethargic and will find a place to curl up and sleep, indicating that the food is in the *kapha* stage of digestion. Once the food goes into the second, or *pitta*-dominant phase, the dog's body temperature rises. He will then get up to look for a drink of water and a cooler, shadier place to sleep. When the food moves into *vata*'s zone in the colon, the dog will suddenly get up, stretch his muscles and go for a walk.

Diagnosis and Transient Phase Metabolism

When we understand the nature of the three phases of *prapaka* digestion, we are better able to identify the specific situations which tend to produce *ama*. The length of time required for food to pass through each phase of transient metabolism is a very important clue as to the source of the digestive problem.

For example, if someone experiences sluggishness until three in the afternoon, after eating at eleven in the morning, it indicates the food is remaining too long in the *kapha* phase of transient metabolism. There are a number of possible explanations for this. First, the food that was eaten was too *kaphic* in nature and has slowed down the digestion. Foods which are excessively sweet, heavy, oily and cold take longer to digest because they require a stronger digestive fire and create more *kapha* as a result. We feel lethargic for a longer period of time after eating heavy, sweet foods. Eating large quantities of food also produce the same effect, as they place a greater demand on *agni*'s ability to digest them.

Second, *kapha* and/or *kapha*-related *ama* could have accumulated in that zone of the body from previous bouts of poor digestion. This excess can either overwhelm or spoil the functions of the other *doshas* there or weaken the digestive fire. The two factors above can then deplete the *agni* or *pitta* function in the second stage of *prapaka* digestion, causing a backup in the first stage.

The source of a digestive problem may also lie in the sour or *pitta* phase of transient digestion. If someone notices increased acidity, even shortly after eating, it shows that sour metabolism has overwhelmed the sweet phase of *prapaka* digestion. This imbalance can also be experienced as more heat and thirst than usual or as a sour or metallic taste in the mouth. A number of factors can account for second stage indigestion. If the digestive *agni* or *pitta* function are normal, then the problem is due to eating too much sour, hot, spicy or fermented food. Adding more heat to an already well-functioning digestive fire can aggravate *pitta*.

A second possible cause is due to an over-accumulation of *pitta* and/or *pitta*-related *ama* that has resulted from past indigestion. This may have occurred due to a weak *agni* which allowed the food to ferment, a prime cause of *pitta*-related *ama*. If *pitta* is too strong, then appetite can be excessive or constant — we might feel hungry an hour or two after eating. Acidity, irritability before eating, and food cravings also indicate *pitta* aggravation.

Problems in the pungent or *vata* stage of transient digestion do not normally occur by themselves. They result from improper metabolism in the two previous phases. This causes either an increase or decrease in pungency which manifests as either constipation or loose bowels. For instance, irritable bowel syndrome is a common problem of *vata* aggravation associated with metabolic deficiencies in the two previous stages.

In general, if the digestive fire is strong, the time it will take to digest our food will be shorter; if it is weak and sluggish, it will take a longer time.

When an Ayurvedic physician is attempting to determine where the source of a patient's indigestion lies, he will often ask his patient the following questions: "How long does it take for you to digest your food?"; "How long do you feel lethargic after eating?"; "Do you become excessively thirsty?" and "When do you become inclined toward activity after eating?" These answers help determine the strength of the patient's digestive fire. The physician can also tell whether *ama* is being produced as a result of weak digestive fire, *doshic* aggravation or unsuitable food. He confirms his findings by feeling the patient's pulse, palpating the abdomen and examining the *malas*. The doctor can then prescribe suitable treatments and recommend dietary changes which will strengthen *agni* and restore normal function to the *doshas*.

Rasa: The Three Types of Taste

A fascinating area of Ayurvedic science is the knowledge of *rasa*, the influence that a food's taste has on digestion. Understanding the three categories of *rasa* can be very helpful in both the diagnosis and treatment of disease. That is why it is important to be able to distinguish between these three types of *rasa* or taste. As was mentioned earlier, the first type of *rasa* is the natural taste of food imparted by the combination of elements that make up that food substance. For example, a food that is high in both *vayu* and *agni* will taste sour and pungent, like chilis or peppers.

The second type of *rasa* is defined by the taste that is acquired by food when it undergoes distinct phases of *prapaka* digestion. As food moves through the G-I tract, it is temporarily converted into a sweet, a sour, and then a pungent taste, reflecting the specific zone or phase of transient metabolism that it is in.

Rasa's third aspect relates to the influence of the food's taste on the post-absorptive or *vipaka* metabolism (which we will be discussing shortly). After a nutrient has undergone *prapaka* digestion, it will often take on a taste that is different either from its original taste or from the taste it took on during any of the various phases of transient digestion. The knowledge of a food's post-digestive taste is utilized by the Ayurvedic physician to influence *vipaka* or *dhatu* metabolism. This influence can be either nourishing or wasting.

For instance, if someone is suffering from emaciation, the physician will prescribe foods with a sweet *vipaka* effect, since the sweet taste is responsible for building tissue in the body. On the other hand, foods with a pungent post-digestive influence have a wasting effect on the *dhatus*. A food's pungent *vipaka* influence can, of course, be very beneficial in situations such as obesity, where it is important to reduce bodily tissue. Knowledge of this third aspect of *rasa* is particularly useful in understanding how various herbal and mineral compounds help to regenerate the *dhatus*.

Ayurveda therefore classifies foods according to both their pre-digestive and post-digestive taste or influence on the body. The knowledge of this area of Ayurvedic science, however, is too detailed to be included in the scope of this book.

VIPAKA METABOLISM: POST-ABSORPTIVE DIGESTION

The process of digestion is not complete when food passes through the three zones of the gastrointestinal tract. The nutrients that result from *prapaka* digestion are still not in a form that can be assimilated by the *dhatus*. Because each *dhatu* has a different structure and function in the body, it requires its own metabolic process — one that can convert the raw nutrients into a form that can be used for its specific nutritional requirements.

Vipaka, or post-absorptive digestion, begins once the nutrients are absorbed into the body from the area surrounding the ileocecal valve, which lies at the juncture of the small and large intestines. This second phase of digestion continues the process of conversion through a fixed sequence of increasingly refined metabolic processes. Each *dhatu* has its own digestive or *dhatu agni*, as distinct from the *jathara agni* operative in the G-I tract. This *agni* converts the raw foodstuffs sent to it from the previous stage of digestion into the precise nutrients needed by that *dhatu*.

Each of the seven *dhatus* gets nourished in the same order that it develops in the body. *Prapaka* digestion converts food into a form that can then be acted upon by *rasa*'s *dhatu agni* and the *doshas*. *Rasa* metabolism, which begins *vipaka* digestion, produces a substance capable of sustaining *rasa dhatu*, the nutrient fluid or plasma. Like a pigeon finding edible grains among pieces of gravel, *rasa* metabolism selects the parts of the processed food-stuff which will nourish it. *Kapha* binds together whatever is unusable and *vata* takes it back to the G-I tract for elimination as *mala*.

Rasa dhatu, however, does not take all nutrients created by its *dhatu agni* for itself. It takes only that portion which is required for its nourishment. The remainder gets bound up by *kapha* and transported by *vata* to *rakta dhatu*'s (blood) metabolic staging ground, which is located primarily in the liver and spleen and, to a lesser degree, in the bone marrow. *Rakta*'s *agni* now transforms the nutrient fluid of *rasa dhatu* into a form that is useful for it. Again, *vata* takes the unusable by-product back to the G-I tract to be discharged as *mala*. *Rakta* keeps a portion of the end-product of this metabolic refinement for its own nourishment. The rest goes to the muscles, the seat of *mamsa dhatu*.

These sorting and transporting mechanisms resemble an irrigation system where water is directed through main and subsidiary channels. Waste products are separated for elimination and the remaining foodstuff continues to the next *dhatu* for further refining until all the *dhatus* have been nourished.

Each *dosha* plays a role in *vipaka* digestion and works in precise coordination with the other two to accomplish this process. As we have indicated, *vata* acts as the carrier vehicle. It takes raw material to the next *dhatu*, separates what is usable and transports both nutrients and waste products to their respective destinations. *Pitta*'s heat converts nutrients into substances that sustain each of the *dhatus*. *Kapha* liquefies and binds the raw food materials, the refined nutrients and the *malas* so that *vata* can then transport them.

Vipaka digestion ends when all the physical substances and structures of the body have received sufficient nourishment. Its final stage takes place in *shukra dhatu* and produces something called *ojas*. *Ojas* represents the essence of the entire digestive process and, according to Ayurveda, is the factor responsible for the body's immunity to disease.

In addition, it is this highly refined biochemical that is responsible for nourishing the non-physical parts of life: the senses, mind and soul. *Ojas* generates harmony and coordination among the four major aspects of human life and establishes their vital connection with *atma* or universal consciousness. It allows every cell in the body to function in direct communication with nature's limitless intelligence. Ultimately, it is this substance that supports the experience of intimate oneness with all of life — enlightenment — the goal of all great spiritual teachings throughout the ages.

Ayurveda places great emphasis on strong, efficient digestion not only because of its vital importance for physical well-being, but also because healthy digestion is vital for connecting the parts of life to their basis in wholeness. Any breakdown in the activities which nourish one *dhatu* will inevitably weaken the health of all the *dhatus* in the developmental sequence. Not only is *ama* produced, but *ojas* becomes depleted and its vital function for life is lost.

Ayurveda's most effective treatment for preventing the formation of *ama* in the first place is education. When we learn how to increase the *sattva* in our minds, we spontaneously make diet and lifestyle choices that truly nourish us and maintain our health and happiness. These choices then ensure that the *doshas* maintain a balanced relationship among themselves and metabolism is efficient. The last part of Chapter Five and the whole of Chapter Six describe the things we can do in our daily routine to increase *sattva* and preserve harmony among the *doshas*.

However, when *ama* is already present in the body, *Panchakarma*, Ayurveda's science of rejuvenation, provides the primary means to re-create health. Through its time-tested purification procedures, *Panchakarma* reestablishes balance among the *doshas*, normalizes digestion and removes the toxic accumulations of *ama* from the *dhatus*. It allows the body's innate healing intelligence to restore the *dhatus* to their normal functioning. *Panchakarma* reverses many cases of degenerative diseases and promotes a long and healthy life. However, its ultimate purpose is to restore the harmonizing function of *ojas* and reestablish our full, conscious connection to universal *atma*, the source of life.

With the knowledge of digestion, we now have a sufficiently firm foundation in Ayurvedic theory to understand how a single system of health can be both comprehensive enough to include all of life and specific enough to address the uniqueness of every individual human being. The next chapter, entitled *Prakruti*, is the culmination of Ayurvedic theory. It gives each person the practical understanding of their uniqueness and how they fit into the cosmic web of life.

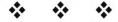

Chapter Five

PRAKRUTI: YOUR UNIQUE CONSTITUTION

$\mathcal{A}$t one time or another, almost everyone has wondered about the vast range of differences that exist among human beings. Though physiologically, we are made of the same substances and function in much the same way, our responses to life vary tremendously. Why do human beings exhibit such diversity in size, shape, complexion, energy levels and health? What produces the great variety in intelligence, emotional responses and adaptability to the environment's demands?

The exact same influences or stimuli seem to produce disparate, even opposite reactions in people. Consequently, we have developed the saying: "One person's food is another person's poison." For example, in a room full of people at a party, some will feel hot and stuffy and want to open a window, while others will feel quite comfortable with the temperature as it is. Still others will feel chilly and want to turn up the heat. What accounts for these diverse experiences of something so simple as room temperature?

It is also common for people to experience the same results from totally opposite influences, as shown in research on longevity. In interviews with the elderly, scientists have not been able to develop a consensus on the factors responsible for a long and healthy life. Some people credit their longevity to working hard and staying busy, while others attribute it to a relaxed, easy-going attitude about life. Some insist that their long life is due to eating a particular type of food, while others claim completely different foods to be responsible for their longevity.

How can we explain the fact that one person eats little, exercises a great deal and still gains weight, while another person gorges on food, rarely exercises and never seems to put on any weight? Why is it that one person can easily handle a hot, spicy, Mexican meal, while another lies awake all night with indigestion? Why does milk nourish and strengthen one individual and give another one stomach cramps, loose bowels or allergies? Why do some people require only five or six hours of sleep, while others need eight or nine hours to feel rested?

Trying to make sense of these differences can be confusing. Few psychological or physiological models of human nature are comprehensive enough to explain the reason behind these differences. As a consequence, no single type of diet, exercise program or medical approach seems to work for everybody.

Your *Doshic* Constitution

However, when the vast array of physical, mental and emotional responses are viewed in light of the theories of *Panchamahabhuta* and *Tridosha*, it all makes perfect sense. As we have already discussed, all phenomena in creation arise from the continuous interaction of the five universal organizing principles or *mahabhutas* and their corresponding physical elements. Though each and every object contains all five elements, there are two factors that account for the vast diversity of physical existence:

   (i) the *bhuta* or *bhutas* that predominate in an object; and

   (ii) the phase of creation (*sattva*, *rajas*, *tamas*) that governs that object.

We are able to gain knowledge of the world — to perceive these ever-changing relationships among the *bhutas* and the *guna*s — because of our minds' ability to compile, compare and discriminate among things. Regardless of whether they are thoughts, feelings or objects within our perceptual field, it is the comparative differences that the mind is able to detect which give us knowledge of diversity. In a field of similarities, nothing stands out. For instance, if all we had ever eaten were strawberries, we would not be able to appreciate their delicious taste. We would never have experienced any other taste with which to compare it.

The differences between things draw our attention and allow us to know them. We watch the Olympics to see which athletes will excel, not to see all the athletes give the same performance. The things within our perceptual field that are most easily known to us are those which stand out — the biggest, the brightest, the loudest, etc. For example, there are many impressively tall mountains that exist in the world, but when asked to name them, most of us remember only one—Mt. Everest. Why? It stands out in our minds as being the tallest.

Vaishamya

The mind's inherent tendency to gain knowledge through comparison and differentiation is what allows us to identify our own particular physiological and psychological predispositions. Just as variations in the physical world exist due to the predominance of one or more *bhutas*, so variations in human beings exist due to the predominance of one or more *doshas*. Our diversity does not arise by chance; it correlates directly with each person's *doshic* make-up.

Each *dosha* displays a unique set of qualities that defines the way it functions in the body. Since it is common for one *dosha*, and sometimes two, to have a predominating influence, its set of qualities or characteristics will be more obvious than those of the other *doshas*. The three, however, are never found in equal dominance. Such a state would destroy the dynamic nature of their relationship and produce a stasis. We would also be unable to perceive any distinctions, since no one set of characteristics would stand out.

This situation never occurs in life. It is the relative disparities among the *doshas* that generates the momentum and change we call evolution. The fact that we can and do identify the differences among ourselves is due to the relative dominance of one or more of the *doshas*.

Each of us is born with a *doshic* "fingerprint," a unique set of traits formed by the relative strengths of the *doshas* in our constitution. Not only our physiology but our personality evolves from this *doshic* make-up. It determines the unique way each of us responds physically, mentally and emotionally. Our dominant *doshic* qualities are like Mt. Everest. The mind recognizes them most easily. This phenomenon is called *vaishamya*. *Vaishamya* is the Ayurvedic term to denote the recognizable influence of one *dosha* over the others, brought about by its predominance in the body.

PRAKRUTI: OUR TRUE NATURE

Ayurveda refers to our *doshic* constitution as *prakruti*, which means "nature." It uses this word to denote both our individual nature and the whole of nature. This underscores the intimate connection which Ayurveda sees existing between the individual and the totality of life.

Knowledge of our *prakruti* permits each of us to recognize our unique style of functioning in the world. When we identify our specific "response-ability," we can optimize our connection to nature by avoiding influences which bring ill-health and unhappiness.

Our *prakruti*, or *doshic* balance, provides a comprehensive understanding of ourselves in relation to the world. It offers an individual profile of the tendencies and predispositions that determine not only our physical functioning but also our mental and emotional characteristics. It includes everything about us: physical structure, complexion, hair color, digestive capacity, appetite and stamina. It describes mental acuity, general personality and emotional reactions. Our *prakruti* defines our truest nature — our most optimal way of being in life. It also describes the ways in which our environment influences us.

Our *prakruti* is determined by the balance of *doshas* with which we are born. For the most part, it is a blend of our parents' *doshic* constitutions at the time of conception. This specific *doshic* balance defines our interactions with the world. The proportion of *dosha(s)* decides our greatest strengths and talents, and when we know our *prakruti*, we can take maximum advantage of them.

When we live life in accord with our innate constitution, our individual nature is perfectly attuned to that of Mother Nature and ideal health results. We excel in our *dharma* (life purpose) and achieve maximum happiness and satisfaction in life with minimum effort.

VIKRUTI: OUR IMBALANCE

Unfortunately, our inborn *doshic* structure often gets distorted or obscured by imbalances. Excessive functioning of our strongest *dosha* constitutes the most common cause of imbalance. When a particular *dosha* is already prominent, it does not take much environmental stimulus to aggravate it. Take, for example, a person with a *pitta prakruti*. *Agni bhuta*—the conversion element— is more prominent in his system than in the systems of people with *vata* or *kapha prakruti*. This gives him a naturally strong digestive fire. However, when he introduces additional heat into the body in the form of hot, spicy food, *pitta* becomes excessive and produces hyperacidity.

The imbalance which obscures the natural, optimum relationship of the *doshas* is called *vikruti*, meaning "out of nature." *Vikruti* arises when there is a predominance of one or more *doshas* that is not natural to our constitution. When this improper relationship exists among the *doshas*, *ama* begins to form which damages the *dhatus* and impairs elimination of the *malas*.

It is important to understand that *vikruti* is a condition which arises from an incorrect relationship with our environment. When we don't know what is best for our particular system, we often expose ourselves to harmful input, such as inappropriate sensory stimuli, improper food and stressful activities. We also make wrong or inadequate adjustments to the impact of seasonal changes. These influences cause physical, mental and emotional stress that overwhelm the system, causing the optimum dynamic relationship among the *doshas* to get distorted. This then compromises our ability to adapt efficiently to life's circumstances.

Prakruti or *Vikruti?*

Two questions naturally arise from the knowledge above. "How do I find out what my *prakruti* is?" and "Should I use *prakruti* or *vikruti* to determine the diet and lifestyle most suitable for my particular constitution?"

These questions have been the source of a great deal of confusion among people interested in the Ayurvedic approach to health and living. The nature of your constitution should be determined by someone experienced in Ayurvedic diagnosis. However, even a highly trained Ayurvedic physician may not be able to ascertain conclusively an individual's constitution in fifteen or twenty minutes. This is because the innate *doshic* predominance is almost always hidden underneath the imbalances caused by years of poor choices in eating and behavior.

If it is so difficult to know our *prakruti* accurately, how do we treat it? The answer is simple. We never have to treat what is most natural to us. We only have to remove that which obscures our true nature. In Ayurveda, all treatment regimens, as well as all dietary and behavioral suggestions, are oriented towards our *vikruti* — pacifying or removing the excesses that create imbalance in the functioning of the *doshas*. As explained previously, these excesses are usually, though not always, related to our strongest *dosha* or *doshas*. When *doshic* aggravation is corrected, the *sattvic* mind's inherent "knowingness" brings to light our *prakruti*, the most advantageous way to relate to life.

The Characteristics of the Three Constitutional Types

In our discussion of the three constitutional types, it is important to keep a number of things in mind. First, just as no one's life ever expresses a perfect balance of all three *doshas*, no one perfectly exemplifies one single *doshic* type. Even though the qualities of the primary *dosha* are most obvious, the characteristics of the less dominant *doshas* always filter through to influence who we are. The degree to which this happens depends on the relative strengths of each *dosha*.

Second, when we look at each *dosha*'s characteristics, our *prakruti* may not be immediately obvious to us. In fact, when we examine lists, charts or tests which help to define our *doshic* makeup, we usually identify with our *vikruti* or imbalances.

Lastly, our most dominant *dosha* is not always responsible for *vikruti* formation. *Vata* can often be the source of imbalance even when it is not the dominant *dosha* because of its pivotal role as the mover in the body. When *vata* gets aggravated, it either pulls the other *doshas* out of balance or causes their excessive activity to travel from their normal sites of activity to other parts of the body. Therefore, Ayurveda places great emphasis on the alleviation of aggravated *vata*.

As we gain familiarity with each *dosha*'s attributes, we recognize their influence more easily. We can facilitate the learning process by recalling the essence of each *dosha*. The *kaphic* constitution is characterized by endurance, increased mass, steadiness and a tendency toward gaining weight. The *pitta*-dominant constitution exhibits strong appetite, sharp intellect and glowing complexion, while the *vata* constitution shows speedy movements, quick mind, thin structure and dry skin. Now let's examine in greater detail the characteristics of each constitutional type as they manifest in both balance and imbalance.

Kapha-Dominant *Prakruti*

Since *kapha dosha* provides the moistening secretions and cohesiveness that nourish the body and provide its bulk, when *kapha* dominates the constitution, a person gains weight relatively easily and the body tends to be thick and bulky. Even when the individual eats well in small amounts and exercises strenuously, body weight is easily maintained.

People with *kaphic* constitutions have relatively slow metabolisms; they take longer to digest their food and they can miss a meal without discomfort. They perform activity in a more leisurely manner, but they have ample strength and stamina and can make sustained efforts without becoming exhausted. Their reactions are slow and even and there is an air of steadiness about them that prevents them from getting easily stressed. All of this leads to a natural resistance to disease.

Kapha people may need a little longer to understand something, but once they understand, they seldom forget. They have good comprehension and good memory. They are even-tempered, content and emotionally stable and are usually satisfied with whatever comes to them. Whether they love or hate, they will hold on to feelings for a long time. *Kapha*'s property of accumulation allows these people to easily gain and maintain both material wealth and loving friends.

Attributes Comparing *Kapha Prakruti* to *Kapha Vikruti*

Kapha Prakruti	Becomes	*Kapha Vikruti*
Provides Nourishment & Bulk to the Body	⟶	Excess Bulk in the Body
Slower Metabolism	⟶	Sluggish Metabolism
Even Tempered Less Expressive Satisfied with Whatever Comes	⟶	Variable in Temper Non-Expressive Non-Reactive

Kapha-Dominant *Vikruti*

When *kapha vikruti* develops, all these favorable qualities get distorted. The individual becomes dull, lethargic, complacent, and becomes apathetic and does not want to move, so much so that he might sleep or rest for abnormally long hours. Digestion is sluggish and he is overweight. The *kaphic* tendency to accumulate changes into possessiveness and greed. People with this imbalance are prone to sinus and respiratory diseases, allergies, obesity, sugar intolerance, indigestion and edema.

Pitta-Dominant *Prakruti*

People with strong *pitta* constitutions show the qualities of heat, sensitivity and intensity associated with both *pitta dosha* and *agni bhuta*. Typically, they are uncomfortable in high temperatures. They prefer cool environments. If given hot food or drinks, they wait for them to cool down before consuming them.

They have big appetites and strong digestion and can digest larger amounts of food than either *kapha* or *vata* types. *Pitta* people have fast metabolisms; they digest food and eliminate wastes quickly. Since their appetite and digestive capacity are strong, when they get too hungry, they may become edgy or irritable. Consequently, they do not tolerate fasting well.

They are usually of medium build with medium strength and stamina. Their skin is soft, warm, reddish and sensitive. *Pitta* types have warm, courageous and loving natures and are quick, witty and intelligent. They are focused, astute and insightful and react quickly to stimuli.

Attributes Comparing *Pitta Prakruti* to *Pitta Vikruti*

Pitta Prakruti	Becomes	*Pitta Vikruti*
Strong Appetite	⟶	Variable Appetite
Strong Metabolism (Digestion)	⟶	Weak Metabolism (Digestion)
Warm, Courageous Intelligent, Sharp Quick-Reactive Soft Skin	⟶	Hot, Angry, Agitated Confusion in Thoughts Impatient, Sensitive Skin Rashes

Pitta-Dominant *Vikruti*

When *pitta* becomes excessive, these types express anger, impatience, irritability and frustration and are also prone to confusion and emotional sensitivity. They are often overly demanding of others and their normally keen intellect and clear speech may develop a sharp and cutting edge. When heat in the body becomes excessive, skin eruptions (rashes and boils), vision problems and baldness may arise. The *pitta vikruti* is prone to acid peptic disorders, liver and gall bladder problems, ulcers, colitis and headaches.

Vata-Dominant *Prakruti*

Since *vata* governs movement and serves a drying function in the body, motility and dryness characterize people with *vata*-dominant constitutions. They exhibit more bodily motion than the other *doshic* types. They move and act quickly but tire easily. Even with ample intake of nutritious food, they have comparatively less stamina. They experience variability in appetite, digestion and elimination.

Their bodies are thin, and either short or tall. Since *vata*'s drying power is stronger than *kapha*'s lubrication, their mouths, nostrils and skin get dry. Dryness is also seen in the relative lack of lubrication of their muscle tissues. This results in less physical strength and stamina than the other types. Their joints may also make a cracking or popping sound because of the low level of lubrication.

Vata people have quick minds and are quick to initiate action. They grasp situations rapidly and make instant decisions. Their responses to life are flexible and they may change their minds and moods frequently.

Attributes Comparing *Vata Prakruti* to *Vata Vikruti*

Vata Prakruti	Becomes	*Vata Vikruti*
Not Much Bulk More Active Gets Tired Easily	⟶	Lose Weight/Structure Hyperactive Always Tired
Quicker Digestion and Elimination	⟶	Sluggish Digestion and Elimination
Quick to Initiate Action Makes Instant Decisions Not Easily Satisfied Dry Skin Cracking in Joints	⟶	Slower in Action; Confusion in Making Decisions; Unsatisfied; Prone to Psychological Problems Very Dry Skin Cold and Stiff Extremities

Vata-Dominant *Vikruti*

People with excessive *vata* experience restlessness and loss of concentration. They are prone to worry, anxiety, confusion and fear, as well as lack of clarity and focus. Sleep can be light or disturbed. *Vata* imbalance produces variable energy levels and fatigue, as well as constipation or erratic bowels, and a tendency to be underweight. Dry skin, stiff joints and cold extremities are common problems. All neurological, psychological and degenerative problems are associated with *vata vikruti*.

Vikruti Specific Questionnaire

Everyone benefits from knowing their *prakruti*, but it is even more beneficial to know your *vikruti*, so that you can address the imbalances which cover your natural constitution. We are therefore providing a list of questions which can help with a preliminary assessment of your *vikruti*. In addition, we recommend that people consult with a fully-trained Ayurvedic expert for confirmation and for advice regarding the best diet and daily and seasonal routine for pacifying their *vikruti*.

The questions below are divided into two sections. The first section relates to mental and emotional characteristics and preferences. The second section concerns physical characteristics. The questions are presented in a multiple choice format with an answer corresponding to each *dosha*: *vata*, *pitta* and *kapha*. For each question, pick the answer that you feel is most applicable to you and put a check mark in that column. It is useful to take this test a number of times, particularly with a person who knows you well. After you complete the questions, total the number of *vata*, *pitta* and *kapha* responses. The totals will give you a good indication of the *dosha* or *doshas* that are out of balance in your constitution.

SECTION I

BEHAVIORAL CHARACTERISTICS

	VATA RESPONSE	*PITTA* RESPONSE	*KAPHA* RESPONSE
1. Performs activity	Very rapidly	With moderate speed	Slowly
2. Motivated, enthusiastic and excitable	Very easily	Moderately	Slowly
3. Moods	Change quickly	Change quickly and intense	Non-changing and steady
4. Learns	Very quickly and easily	Somewhat quickly and easily	Slowly
5. Quality of mind	Quick, creative and imaginative but restless	Sharp, penetrating intellect	Stable
6. Memory	Good short–term	Medium	Good long-term
7. Digestion	Inconsistent, varies between weak and strong	Usually strong	Weak, slow
8. Appetite	Variable, can skip meals occasionally	Strong, consistent appetite, not comfortable skipping meals	Usually mild, can skip meals without discomfort
9. Quantity of food eaten	Variable	Likes large meals	Likes small meals
10. Taste preferences	Sweet, sour and salty	Sweet, bitter and astringent	Pungent, bitter and astringent
11. Thirst	Varies	Frequent	Very rarely
12. Food preferences	Warm, moist foods	Cool foods	Warm, dry foods

115

13. Drink preferences	Hot	Cold	Hot
14. Frequency of bowel movement	Irregularly	Two or more times a day	Regularly,
15. Consistency of feces	Hard, dry stools	Loose stools soft stools	Well-formed,
16. Perspiration	Moderate	Profuse with body odor	Slight
17. Sexual desire	Small	Small to moderate	Abundant
18. Amount of sleep	Usually 5-6 hours	Usually 6-8 hours	Usually 8 hours or more
19. Quality of sleep	Light, easily interrupted	Deep and uninterrupted	Deep and heavy
20. Type of dreams	Fear, flying, running, jumping, climbing trees and mountains	Anger, violence, struggle, war; fire, lightning, the sun; gold and light	Water, lakes, rivers, oceans; clouds, swans, flowers and romance
21. Response to challenge	Uncertain, worried and indecisive	Angered, irritable and impatient	Clear, stable and patient
22. Speech	Fast, omitting words and digressing	Fast, clear and precise	Slow, clear and sweet
23. Gait	Fast, with a light step	Medium speed, with precise, determined step	Slow, steady and fluid

SECTION II

PHYSICAL CHARACTERISTICS

	VATA RESPONSE	*PITTA* RESPONSE	*KAPHA* RESPONSE
1. Shape of face	Thin, bony, and elongated, plain looking	Oval, angular with medium fullness	Round, full and attractive
2. Complexion	Dark, brownish or black	Fair, reddish or coppery	Light, clear and whitish
3. Involuntary bodily movements	Twitching, jerking and fine tremors	Body is usually still still	Body is usually
4. Body weight	Light; five to ten pounds below normal	Normal; medium weight	Heavy; five or more pounds above normal
5. Build	Lean, thin, tall or short	Medium build, medium height	Thick, large, fleshy or plump
6. Texture or quality of skin	Dry, coarse, rough, cracked or scaling and birthmarks	Soft, delicate and sensitive with freckles, moles	Soft, smooth, and oily
7. Skin moistness	Dry	Moist and slightly oily	Oily
8. Body temperature	Low; cold extremities	High; always, feels warm	Low; body feels cool
9. Stamina	Short	Moderate	Strong
10. Shape and quality of eyes and lashes	Small, bulging, and deep-set with thin, scanty eye lashes	Sharp, intense and penetrating with brown, blond or coppery lashes	Large, attractive and full with long thick lashes

11. Dominant hue of sclera	Dark	Yellow or reddish	White, glossy
12. Peculiar characteristics of eyes	Dry; frequent blinking	Light-sensitive; easily reddened	Teary or runny
13. Teeth	Very small or protruding, crooked; easily cracked	Moderate size, yellowish	Strong and large; white
14. Nails	Short, rough brittle, dark and lusterless	Slightly oily; coppery or pink in color	Long, thick, and well-rooted; soft, glossy and white
15. Lips	Dark, dry and cracked	Soft, pink or copper-colored	Full, thick, moist and oily
16. Size and shape of fingers	Very short or very long; stubby and thick	Medium length, square or oval-shaped	Medium length, elegantly shaped
17. Color and texture of hair	Thin, coarse, dry and wiry; darker in color or balding	Thin, fine, soft blond or red; early graying	Thick, glossy. firmly-rooted, wavy and black
18. Body hair	Scanty	Moderate	Thick and plentiful
19. Joints	Loose or rigid; pronounced; crack and pop	Smooth, flexible well knit;	Strong, well hidden
20. Veins	Prominent or branching; close to surface	Neither hidden nor prominent	Deep and hidden

21. Chest	Long, sunken; thin ribs easily visible	Medium in length medium thick, ribs not so visible	Broad, strong and covered with flesh or fat
22. Body odor	Little or no smell or perspiration	Strong; armpits smell fetid	None
23. Tongue	Dark, brownish, thick, rough and very cracked on the sides	Pink or dark red; soft and long	Light pink, heavy and moist

Now, count the number of *vata*, *pitta* and *kapha* responses in both sections. The *dosha* with the greatest number of points shows your *vikruti*. Since your *vikruti* is generally your overused, dominant *dosha*, this test provides a rough indication of your *prakruti* as well.

Sometimes two *doshas* receive the same (or close to the same) number of responses. This means that you have a *dwandaj* or two-*dosha vikruti*. This is quite common and demands that both *doshas* be considered when you tailor your diet and lifestyle. Which of the two receives the most emphasis will vary according to the seasons. However, always keep in mind that *vata* drives the other *doshas*. If it received a score as high as another *dosha*'s, Ayurveda advises you to first pacify *vata*.

Conclusion

Keep in mind that all three *doshas* are always present and functioning in everyone. Diet, lifestyle, climate and stage of life all affect how strongly a person displays the characteristics associated with his individual constitution.

Prakruti influences every area of life, including all natural preferences and aversions. Personal constitution also affects susceptibility to illness and the types of illness to which someone is prone. A person who is rarely ill most likely is *kapha*-dominant. If someone gets sick easily, this usually indicates *vata*-dominance. For *pitta* people, the incidence of illness generally falls somewhere in between the two.

Whatever our *doshic* make-up, we are predisposed to utilize our strongest qualities excessively. With proper awareness of these tendencies, we can use the right diet and lifestyle choices to counteract aggravation of our main *dosha*. Correct food and behavior provide the keys to compensate for innate tendencies towards illness. No matter what our constitution, these things allow us to maintain and enhance our health.

FOOD PREFERENCES

People naturally prefer foods which balance the excessive influence of their primary *dosha*. For example, *kaphic* people normally shun rich, oily, cold and sweet foods, as well as dairy products, because these foods augment the already excessive action of *kapha* in their bodies. Instead, they choose dry, porous and light foods, like puffed grains, crackers, toast and salads. Because dry foods have greater absorptive capacity, they reduce the abundance of moistening and cohesive secretions that are typical of the *kaphic* nature. *Kaphic* individuals like warm food and enjoy and benefit from spices and pungent condiments. Pungent foods and fasting counteract excessive *kapha*, and these people are usually comfortable missing a meal or fasting.

Contrast this with people having *vata* constitutions. These types enjoy foods that are rich in cream, oils, butter and *ghee* because these substances counterbalance *vata*'s drying effect. They naturally prefer food and drink that is hot, oily and nourishing, and have a spontaneous aversion for dry, toasted and porous foods which aggravate the already dry state of their bodies. Fasting does not suit *vata* people because it decreases their stamina. The constant movement that is typical of a *vata* constitution requires frequent replenishment of food and water in order to maintain its energy level.

Dominant *pitta* gives people a strong digestive *agni*, faster metabolism and more heat in their bodies. As a result, they like large meals and cool foods and drinks. If given a cup of hot tea or soup, they wait until it cools down before drinking it. Many *pitta* people have an aversion to alcoholic beverages, because the hot, pungent nature of alcohol aggravates *pitta* and can produce nausea, gastritis and ulcers.

People do not always choose foods that balance their dominant *dosha*. When a person's system is grossly out of balance, they actually develop food and behavior preferences that exacerbate their condition. When *vikruti* covers over or distorts their inherent "knowingness" to such a degree, they become prone to food cravings and addictions.

Identifying The *Doshic* Predominance In Food

It is not always possible to carry around a list that tells us which foods will pacify or aggravate which *doshas*. It is much more practical to be able to identify foods based on their qualities, and to know how these qualities either augment or decrease our primary *dosha*. We should know that foods which increase *vata* exhibit cold, dry, rough, hard and light qualities. Foods which are hot, sharp, oily and light increase *pitta*, while those that are cold, heavy, liquid and unctuous elevate *kapha*.

For example, let's compare the qualities of a banana and a watermelon. Both taste sweet, but significant differences cause us to recognize the banana as *kapha*-promoting and the watermelon as *vata*-enhancing. When we cut or crush a banana, water does not separate from its mass; the substance coheres and holds onto its water content. The banana has a heavy and unctuous character which reflects its *kaphic* nature. However, if we cut or crush a piece of watermelon, it immediately gives up its water content. It is primarily *vata* and not particularly substantial. One-quarter pound of banana will provide strength and nourishment to the body; the same amount of watermelon does not provide much nourishment. Instead, it has a diuretic effect; it dries the body and augments *vata*.

Dosha Augmenting Foods

Grains (Wheat, Rice, Millet) Fruit (Banana) Dairy Product	Increases *Kapha Dosha*
Spices (Cayenne, Pepper, Turmeric, Chilli)	Increases *Pitta Dosha*
Staple Foods Legumes	Increases *Vata Dosha*

As another example, we can compare grains and legumes. Wheat, rice, millet and similar grains remain in their hulls even when they are fully matured and dried. They have a heaviness and wetness or oiliness that does not allow moisture to separate from the solid particles. Their *kaphic* nature makes them nourishing, tissue-building and lubricating. By contrast, when legumes like beans and lentils mature, they dry out, crack open and fall out of their pods. Unlike grains, which are directly tissue-building, these *vata*-dominant beans and lentils provide energy and motility for the body.

Pitta-dominant, *pitta*-augmenting food substances are brightly colored — red, yellow or greenish. They appear shiny and bright and are much lighter in weight than *kaphic* foods. They have a strongly spicy, sour or pungent flavor. Cayenne pepper, turmeric, ginger powder, chilies and tamarind provide common examples. When used in moderation, they improve metabolism, but when taken to excess, they create too much heat in the body.

Even these few illustrations show how it is possible to predict the effect that certain foods will have on the body. If a food retains its moisture content and resists disintegration, it is likely to increase *kapha*. If it is brightly colored, shiny, lightweight, spicy, pungent or salty, it probably increases *pitta*. If it easily loses water content, dries out and cracks open by itself, or is porous, hard and rough, it augments *vata*.

Treating *Vikruti* With Diet

Using these general guidelines, we can select foods that compensate for constitutional tendencies towards *doshic* excess. For instance, since *vata* is rough, dry, hard, light and cold, foods like crackers, with the same characteristics, only increase *vata*. We can counterbalance the qualities of *vata* with foods that are warm, moist, oily and heavy foods that are also generally sweet, sour and salty. Someone with *vata vikruti* should favor moist, lubricating, nutritive and tissue-building foods, which compensate for high *vata*. *Vata*-balancing foods include *ghee*, butter, dairy products, bananas, wheat, rice, barley and corn.

Pitta's hot, sharp, oily and light properties can be counterbalanced with foods that display cool, dry and heavy qualities. These foods taste sweet, bitter and astringent. A *pitta* constitution should avoid sour, pungent or salty foods and does better with foods and drinks which are cooler, but not cold. These include milk, butter, *ghee*, most fruits, rice and barley.

Doshas Pacified by Tastes

Vata Dosha	Sweet, Sour, Salty
Pitta Dosha	Sweet, Bitter, Astringent
Kapha Dosha	Pungent, Bitter, Astringent

We can offset *kapha*-dominance by eating a smaller quantity of food and by eating foods which exhibit more *vata*. The cold, heavy, liquid and dull nature of *kapha* can be counterbalanced with foods that are hot, light, dry and sharp, or those that taste bitter, pungent and astringent. Foods that are dry and light and have pungent and astringent tastes counteract *kapha*'s tendency toward excess secretions and sluggishness by adding *vata*'s dryness and motility. Such foods include puffed wheat, rice and corn. The puffing process removes the liquid and creates lightness and dryness. Light, dry grains like rye, millet, amaranth, couscous and quinoa also offset surplus *kapha*.

As we become familiar with the essential characteristics of each *dosha*, we'll gain an intuitive feeling for identifying which foods can correct our *vikruti*.

VIKRUTI PACIFYING DIETS

Each *vikruti* responds favorably to a particular diet. The items listed below constitute the most ideal foods to reduce the excessive influence of the corresponding *dosha*. The more closely you can follow the diet recommended for your *vikruti*, the more quickly your *prakruti*, or ideal constitutional balance, will become apparent. However, don't strain on any diet. Gently favor the foods that are good for you, and eat less often the foods that fuel your *vikruti*. As *vikruti* disappears and more balance is established, it becomes easier to make life-supporting food choices; the innate ability to recognize beneficial foods — your "knowingness" — becomes more and more available to *sattvic* minds.

Vata Pacifying Food List

Grains	white and brown *basmati* rice, wheat, barley, amaranth, oats and quinoa
Legumes	mung beans, aduki beans, split yellow mung *dal*, red and yellow split pea and urad *dal*. All these should be cooked to a soft consistency
Fruits	sweet and sour tastes, like grapes, lemons, pears, bananas, sweet oranges, dates, figs, apples (preferably cooked), avocados, berries and a small amount of raisins
Vegetables	sweet vegetables, like zucchini, beets, cauliflower, leeks, carrots, asparagus, cilantro, fennel and a small amount of garlic, green beans, green chilies, okra, parsnips, pumpkins and radishes (preferably cooked)
Spices	Avoid using hot, pungent, drying spices. Use fresh spices like ginger root, cilantro, cumin, coriander and fennel seeds, turmeric and asafoetida (hing)
Dairy	fresh, whole, unhomogenized milk, *ghee* and a small amount of butter
Meats	white meat, like chicken, fish or turkey (baked or broiled), and chicken broth
Nuts	a small amount of almonds, pecans and sesame seeds
Oils	*ghee*, sesame and olive in a smaller amount

Pitta Pacifying Food List

Grains	white and brown *basmati* rice, barley, oat bran, oats, wheat and wheat bran
Legumes	yellow mung *dal*, split red and yellow peas, a small amount of aduki beans and soy products. All these should be cooked to a soft consistency
Fruits	sweet fruits, such as apples, berries, coconuts, dates, figs, avocados, sweet melons, plums and pomegranates
Vegetables	asparagus, broccoli, cabbage, cucumber, cooked onions, sweet potatoes, sprouts, squash and a small amount of okra and cauliflower
Spices	cooling spices, like licorice, cardamom, coriander seeds, cilantro, fennel seeds, fresh basil, dill, turmeric and a small amount of cumin and fresh ginger
Dairy	fresh *ghee* and fresh, whole unhomogenized milk
Meats	baked or broiled chicken, turkey or white fish in moderate amounts
Nuts	sunflower seeds and almonds in moderate amounts
Oils	coconut, sunflower, canola and a small amount of sesame

Kapha Pacifying Food List

Grains	barley, buckwheat, couscous, millet, muesli, oats, oat bran and a small amount of wheat
Legumes	most beans, peas and *dal*. Avoid soy products
Fruits	apples, berries, cranberries, pomegranates, dried fruits and a small amount of strawberries
Vegetables	asparagus, beets, bitter melons, broccoli, beet greens, cabbage, garlic, green beans, fennel, carrot, kale, horseradish, leafy greens, leeks, lettuce, okra, cooked onions, spinach, sprouts, squash, turnip and a small amount of artichoke, burdock root and brussel sprouts
Spices	hot spices, like pepper, chilies, ginger, cinnamon, clove, fenugreek and bay leaves
Dairy	a very small amount of dairy; goat milk and *ghee* in moderation
Meats	freshwater fish, shrimp, rabbit, venison, and a small amount of the white meat of chicken and turkey
Nuts	a small amount of almonds
Oils	a small amount of olive, corn and canola

Nutritional Guidelines for All *Vikrutis*

If you are having some difficulty in determining your *vikruti* and a diet to reduce it, the following diet restores balance to all constitutions and prevents *ama* from being formed. Whenever possible, eat organic foods. Base your diet on four food groups: grains, beans, vegetables and fruits:

Tridosha Balancing Food List

Grains	white and brown *basmati* rice, millet, quinoa, barley
Legumes	mung *dal*, yellow mung *dal*, red lentils, aduki
Fruits	cooked apple, pear, papaya, black raisins, banana, mango and oranges in moderation. Always eat fruit by itself
Vegetables	spinach, zucchini, broccoli, cauliflower, cabbage, asparagus, sweet potatoes, carrots, leafy greens. Steam, boil, bake or stir-fry the vegetables
Salads	fresh, green salad with sesame oil and lemon juice dressing and spices of choice
Spices	fresh ginger root, turmeric, coriander seeds and leaves, cumin seeds, licorice, fennel seeds, cardamom, cinnamon, fresh basil, mustard seeds and hing (asafoetida)
Salts	in moderation mineral salts, black salt or rock salt
Sweeteners	in moderation uncooked honey, maple syrup, sucanat (dried sugarcane juice)
Nuts and Seeds	in moderation blanched almonds, unsweetened coconut, sesame and pumpkin seeds
Oils	*ghee*, sesame, olive, sunflower, flax seed, canola
Breads	unleavened, unfermented breads, wheat and corn tortillas and chappatis
Beverages	warm herbal teas or grain beverages, plenty of water (unrefrigerated)

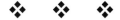

Chapter Six

AHARA, VIHARA AND AUSHADHI: THE THREE PILLARS OF AYU

The purpose of this book up until now has been to lay the conceptual foundation for understanding how this "science of life" can create ideal health. On this firm foundation, we can now construct the "pillars of *ayu*," the basic principles upon which health, happiness and harmony with natural law rest. These three pillars are referred to as *ahara*, *vihara* and *aushadhi*.

The first two of these supports, *ahara* and *vihara*, are concerned with diet and lifestyle and are fundamentally preventative in nature. When their principles are followed, the seeds of disease never get sown. They serve to educate us how to live life in harmony with natural law. The practical, easy to follow guidelines which *ahara* and *vihara* provide, assist us in bringing out the fullness of our life. When our *prakruti* is obscured by our *vikruti*, these dietary and behavioral recommendations will go a long way to bring balance back to our lives.

The imbalances that cannot be handled by these two pillars are managed by *aushadhi*, whose concern is treatment of disease. This third support of health translates literally as "medicine" and implies the various treatments that Ayurveda prescribes to bring us back to health. Since the entire second half of this book is devoted to the principles of *aushadhi*, this chapter will concentrate on the fundamentals of *ahara* and *vihara*.

AHARA: LIFE-SUPPORTING DIET

Ahara, the first pillar, means "intake" and refers to the knowledge of proper diet. It provides the first approach we can take to create and maintain ideal health and to alleviate the symptoms of illness. While diet will not cure well-established diseases, sixty percent of illnesses can be controlled solely by adjustments in diet and eating habits. Since diet is such a significant aspect of maintaining good health, we should be aware of what, when and how we are eating. If our eating habits are not conducive to health, we must be willing to make the changes necessary to stop the formation of new *ama*.

These changes entail eating to counteract our *vikruti*, or *doshic* imbalance. The last chapter gave an extensive list of foods that are *dosha*-specific, to help you determine a diet that is most appropriate for your particular constitutional type. In this chapter, we provide knowledge of the deleterious effects of certain foods as well as some general dietary guidelines which reduce the burden on the digestive fire, increase *sattva* in the mind and help alleviate symptoms of digestive dysfunction. These guidelines are valuable for everyone, regardless of their *vikruti*.

Ayurvedic Nutrition

The Ayurvedic understanding of nutrition is quite different from that of the West. The primary focus of Western nutrition is on the physical attributes of food: the amount of protein, fat, carbohydrates, vitamins and minerals. *Ahara*, on the other hand, is concerned with the effects of various types of food on the quality of the mind, the digestion and the balance of the *doshas*. As discussed earlier, Ayurveda asserts that almost all diseases arise on a physical level from improper metabolism, and generally attributes this to weak digestive *agni* and imbalanced *doshic* functioning. Ayurveda also recognizes the crucial role proper nutrition plays in maintaining mental *sattva* — the key to keeping the parts of life fully connected to their underlying source in wholeness.

Role of Taste in Nutrition

In Chapter Four, we alluded to the role that taste plays in both *prapaka* and *vipaka* digestion, the metabolic processes that create and maintain the *dhatus*. Complete nutrition requires that all six tastes be available in our daily diet, indicating that all five *bhutas* are present in the necessary proportions in our food. Because *jala* and *prithvi bhutas* are found in the greatest proportion in the body, the sweet taste associated with them is required in greater amounts for its strengthening and nourishing qualities.

To understand how food affects us, we must recognize that all five elements are present in the foods we eat and in the body's organs and tissues. Governed by the *doshas*, digestion transforms food into substances suitable to the unique elemental composition of the various tissues and organs of the body. Like increases like. Food that is high in one *bhuta* increases the *dosha* which represents that *bhuta* in the body. For example, if we eat food dominated by *prithvi* and *jala*, it increases *kapha* and decreases *akash* and *vayu*, or *vata dosha*. Food high in *agni* increases *pitta* and decreases *kapha*.

Ayurveda uses taste to determine which elements are high in each food. The six basic tastes arise out of the various combinations and permutations of the five elements. As a result, certain tastes increase the influence of one *dosha* and decrease the effects of the other two. Since the elemental make-up of food can aggravate or excite a *dosha*, foods are categorized according to the tastes which pacify or decrease a *dosha*'s aggravation.

When we know the effect of tastes on the *doshas*, we can select foods which keep the *doshas* balanced and create optimum digestion. All three *doshas* must be nourished and this is accomplished by taking in all six tastes in the appropriate proportions on a daily basis. A diet habitually unbalanced in taste creates *doshic* disorders and *ama*. For instance, if we eat only sweet, sour and salty foods, *vata* gets nourished but *pitta* and *kapha* do not. This throws off the natural equilibrium that exists among the three of them.

The proper balance of tastes is slightly different for every individual. An appropriate diet takes both *prakruti* and *vikruti* into account. Such a diet can correct current imbalances by pacifying the excessive *doshas* and strengthening the weak ones. In this way it can bring us back into harmony with our true "nature." Chapter Five has already provided a detailed understanding of the effects of food on *doshic* balance.

Let's now look at the ways in which different foods affect both the quality of the mind and the body's ability to convert them into substances capable of nourishing the *dhatus*. We start with an analysis of modern methods of food production and their consequences.

Microwaving & Genetic Engineering

Ayurveda states that humankind is part of nature. Therefore, any time nature is altered, the effects of that alteration will express itself directly in humanity. In modern man's attempt to create convenience (microwave), produce food which is not vulnerable to the elements or insects, and has a longer shelf life, etc., (genetic engineering), there will be serious repercussions which, over time, the body may express through sluggish metabolism.

The Effects of Processed Foods

This century has transformed the ways in which food is prepared and presented to the consumer. Because of the rapid pace of life and the trend towards urbanization, we have less access to fresh food and less time to prepare it. As a result, we have become more and more dependent on packaged, processed food. Though this has added convenience to life, it has had a deleterious effect on physical and mental health.

Due to the high incidence of arterial and coronary diseases in the West, laws have been passed making it mandatory for manufacturers to list the contents of processed foods, particularly the amount of fat, sodium and carbohydrates. However, these labels do not inform us of the negative impact from the methods used to produce, process and preserve the food. From the Ayurvedic perspective, these considerations are extremely important in determining whether food is healthy or not. Let's look at the consequences of various aspects of modern food production for the mind, digestion and *doshic* balance.

Chemicals in Food Production

Most of today's food, whether it is meat or vegetables, is grown with artificial fertilizers, hormones, antibiotics, herbicides and pesticides. Because of the synthetic or inorganic nature of these substances, the body has great difficulty metabolizing them and, as a result, they produce a toxic residue which blocks the *shrotas*. This prevents nutritive substances from reaching the *dhatus*; in addition, these poisonous substances damage the *dhatus* themselves.

Foods derived from the killing of animals may give physical energy and strength, but they have a harmful side effect. At the time of death, the animal experiences both fear and anger — the same emotions we would experience if our lives were threatened. Science is now starting to discover that every emotion has a corresponding biochemical within the body which translates that emotional reaction into a physical response. The chemicals in the meat that are associated with fear and anger trigger the "fight or flight" response in our system, which stimulates the production of adrenaline and other stress hormones. This response strains the system, and when activated often enough, creates wear and tear on the body and eventually decreases the immune system's ability to perform its job.

The anger-producing influence of meat also aggravates *pitta*, because anger is a hot emotion. Since meat is such a heavy substance to digest, it also greatly taxes *agni*'s capacity to metabolize it. The effects of eating red meat are borne out in the latest research which shows that meat-eaters are more prone to heart disease, various degenerative diseases and cancer. Finally, from the perspective of mental health, the anger and fear in meat create *rajas* and *tamas* in the mind, overshadowing *sattva* and clouding our experience of "knowingness."

Freezing

Time is at a premium in Western countries, creating a habit of cooking one large meal and freezing the leftovers. When the food is defrosted, a new meal is available without much additional trouble. Though the defrosted food looks and tastes pretty much the same, and has the same components of fat, carbohydrates and protein, it has a very different influence on the body and mind than fresh food. Refrigerated or frozen food can no longer enliven the *sattvic* quality in the mind nor truly nourish the body. It has lost its essential vitality.

Ayurveda calls any food which has been left overnight, *paryushit*, or "lifeless food." To illustrate this point, notice what happens when you defrost food and set it beside the same food in fresh form. The defrosted food decomposes much more quickly, taking on a dried, colorless look, and starts to give off a putrid odor after a short time, indicating *vata* dominance.

When we eat fresh food, we take in and assimilate its orderly structure. This nourishes us and increases orderliness in our own structure. When we eat old or defrosted food, we consume substances that have already been subjected to the disorganizing effects of entropy. We essentially ingest disorder and, as the saying goes: "We are what we eat." When we take in disorder, it generates a disorganizing influence in the body. Rather than promote proper tissue formation through the production of refined endproducts, it accelerates *dhatu* degeneration by creating unmetabolized precursors of disease.

In addition, food that has been subjected to cold develops a heavy, *kaphic* quality which puts a strain on our digestive fire, thus further impeding the ability of the metabolic processes to assimilate any remaining orderliness or nutritive value that may be left in the food. *Agni* always prefers to work on food substances that are at body temperature or slightly warmer.

What we are discussing here are the basic laws of thermodynamics as they manifest in the body. The third law of thermodynamics states that a system can maintain its orderly structure and prevent the disintegrating effects of entropy — described by the second law — only if order is constantly introduced.

Ayurveda is not against the principle of refrigeration, which helps to preserve food. It does caution against eating cold foods or drinks or leftover cooked foods. Applying *agni* to any food accelerates the transformation process, speeding up the movement of the food towards disintegration. If we do not eat food soon after cooking, it loses its *dhatu*-building ability because it goes quickly into the third, or *vata*, stage of transient metabolism. If the food that we eat is already in the pungent phase, it can only have a degenerative effect on the body. Refrigeration cannot impede this process in already cooked food.

A final but very important point in this regard is that the quality of *tamas* dominates old or lifeless food. *Tamas* creates a thick veil of dullness and inertia over the mind, intellect and senses, which obscures our ability to see and choose what is good for us, impairing the functions of *dhi*, *dhriti*, and *smriti* discussed in Chapter One.

Chemical Preservation

Food which is preserved chemically has essentially the same effect as food preserved by freezing. However, it has the added harmful influence of the synthetic chemicals used to retard spoilage.

Raw Foods

The emphasis on fresh food inevitably brings up the question of eating raw as opposed to cooked food. Some people in the West believe that it is much healthier to have a diet composed mainly of salads and uncooked vegetables. The argument in favor of eating raw foods states that the process of cooking destroys food's natural enzymes, vitamins and minerals. Ayurveda, on the other hand, asserts that the potential of these nutrients is not actually available to the body until *agni* is applied in the form of heat. The conversion process that takes place during cooking saves the *agni* in the *pitta* zone of the body from having to work so hard to make the nutritive components in the vegetables available to the *dhatus*.

Chapter Four discussed the physiological roles of *agni* and *pitta*. *Agni* has a general conversion function, whereas *pitta* has a more specific role. It supplies the necessary digestive secretions to metabolize food. When *agni* is weak, *pitta*'s digestive ability decreases. With raw foods, we also have to expend more energy in mastication in order to supply increased *kapha* secretions to ingest the dry, raw foods. This increases *vata* by exhausting the *kapha* function. Consequently, in the end, raw foods offer relatively less energy and nutritive substance for the body's post-absorptive metabolic processes than cooked foods.

In addition, the hard, rough and cold qualities of raw foods increase *vata*. People whose diet consists primarily of raw foods show a higher incidence of *vata* aggravation, evidenced by dry, rough skin, some slight emaciation, often scattered, unfocused mental capacity or weakened digestive capacity. These symptoms are more pronounced in people who already have *vata vikruti*.

This does not mean that raw foods should be eliminated from our diet, but in general, they should not compose more than a quarter of our food intake. Obesity or excess *kapha*, however, constitute an exception to this rule. In these situations, the separating or wasting influence in raw foods makes them beneficial.

Fermentation

Fermentation provides a popular way of flavoring food. Our everyday diet includes many fermented foods, such as vinegar, alcohol, soy sauce, yogurt, cheese, yeasted breads and crackers, pickles and ketchup. The dictionary defines fermentation as a chemical transformation with effervescence, or the transformation of an organic substance by agitation or intense activity. Both these definitions indicate that *vata*, or motion, has a more pronounced influence in fermented substances.

Chapter Four explained that *vata*'s disintegrating force dominates the third stage of *prapaka* digestion, where bubbles are created as water separates from solid substance. In fermented foods, the disintegration process has started even before we eat them. When we ingest this type of food, it disturbs the sweet and sour phases of *prapaka* digestion, and aggravates the pungent phase as well. As was mentioned above, *vata* has a separating influence which both prevents proper tissue formation and produces tissue degeneration. This knowledge shows why tissue degeneration or emaciation is one of the most pronounced effects of alcohol abuse.

Fermented foods are also considered *paryushit* — "lifeless food," and as a result, create *tamas* or dullness in the mind. Again, alcohol offers a good example of the effects of fermented substances on the quality of the mind. Alcohol produces weak, faulty cognition, dulls the senses, slows down physical responses and impairs coordination.

In a number of research studies in India, laboratory animals were fed *sattvic*, *rajas*ic and *tamas*ic foods. When they were given fresh, mostly vegetarian food, they became calm, alert and lively. However, when they ate leftover foods, frozen foods and non-vegetarian foods, they became restless and violent. *Charaka* wrote thousands of years ago that too much *rajas* and *tamas* weakens digestion and creates illness. We can verify for ourselves the influence of various kinds of food in our lives. When we avoid old, fermented, excessively pungent foods, we will see how digestion improves, the mind and senses become clear, and peace and calmness settle into our lives.

Refined Foods

Manufacturers alter the nature of the food and improve its appearance, flavor or texture through yet another method — refinement. In this process, the fibrous covering is separated from the food. We see this most often in the refinement of wheat, rice and sugar. Removing the roughage diminishes food's holistic benefits. The fiber surrounding the nutritive component is essential for peristalsis in the colon. Constipation is one of the most common outcomes of eating refined foods.

The refining process yields end-products which are small and highly potent, and which accelerate the movement of *vata*. As a result, *agni* does not have time to metabolize them before they are assimilated. Rather than nourish the *dhatus*, these substances promote disintegration.

Refined sugar illustrates this well. Unlike unprocessed sugar-cane juice, which contains many minerals and nutrients, refined sugar quickly passes undigested through *rasa* and *rakta* metabolism, immediately overloading the liver, pancreas and other organs of the *pitta* zone. Its light, refined quality increases pungency which generates fermentation. This then increases acidity and quickly consumes the body's minerals and other nutrients.

Children who eat too much refined sugar (candies, chocolate, cookies, etc.) become hyperactive for some time after eating these foods, showing the influence of excessive *vata*. Studies also indicate that over-consumption of sweets and chocolate produce a long-term depletion of calcium in the bones, one of *vata*'s seats. Teeth provide an obvious manifestation of bone formation, and high levels of sugar consumption have been directly correlated with tooth decay.

Fried Foods

Frying is another popular way to prepare food. Though this process enhances taste, the oil in the food makes it heavy and difficult to digest because it taxes *agni*'s ability to metabolize it. Fried food produces an acidic residue in the stomach which creates hyperacidity. The resulting increase in heat also generates a *rajas*ic influence in the mind, as do any hot, spicy substances. In addition, deep-fried foods promote *tamas* in the mind due to the heaviness arising from the large amount of oil used in cooking.

Additives, Colorings and Flavorings

Unfortunately, food manufacturers commonly enhance the taste and appearance of food through the use of artificial flavors and colors. These substances are as indigestible as all the other synthetic chemicals used in food production and preservation. They deplete *agni* and poison the body.

Sugar and Salt

Much of the processed food we eat is heavily salted or sweetened. Sugar and salt not only improve the flavor but act to preserve the food; bacteria cannot live in high concentrations of either sugar or salt. A little bit of sugar or salt improves *rasa* metabolism and pacifies *vata*. However, when taken in excess, they have a toxic effect on the system. Too much sugar aggravates *kapha* and increases *rajas* and over time, creates mental *tamas*. Too much salt aggravates *pitta* and produces *rajas*.

Hot, Spicy Food

Spices play an important role in food preparation. They augment *pitta* secretions in the body's mid-zone, helping *pitta* to metabolize food efficiently. However, in the modern diet, many foods have such a high concentration of spices that they produce the opposite influence on digestion. The amount of heat in foods like pizza, Mexican food, barbecue sauces, pickles, mustard, etc., generates *pitta* imbalances, which create indigestion. These spicy foods also significantly increase mental *rajas*, which makes us feel restless and agitated.

Carbonation

A significant number of people in Western societies take a large percentage of their fluids in the form of carbonated beverages. The carbonation process injects carbon dioxide into flavored, sweetened water. This gives the drink a refreshing quality and enhances its taste, but the effervescence generates intense activity, which vitiates *vata* and produces hyperactivity in the G-I tract. This impedes absorption and assimilation and creates *rajas* in the mind as well.

Food Allergies

Many people are now starting to develop allergies to specific foods, particularly wheat and dairy. However, from the Ayurvedic point of view, the foods are not the culprits. The source of the problem lies in the way they are processed, preserved and presented. Let's take milk as an example. When milk is homogenized, it is subjected to a process that augments *vata*. In addition, preserving it through refrigeration and serving it cold greatly increases milk's already *kaphic* influence. This heaviness creates a burden on the digestive fire, which ultimately weakens its ability to digest the milk. Food allergies are symptoms caused by the body's inability to digest those particular foods. Sinus and respiratory problems, as well as skin conditions, comprise some of the many manifestations of food allergies.

Fresh, Whole Foods

When we eat fresh foods which are naturally sweet, while blending all six tastes, our bodies get deeply nourished, our intellects grow sharper and our memories improve. Natural foods, prepared from fresh ingredients, are easy to digest and amplify the *sattvic* quality of the mind. When *sattva* dominates, it's simple to live in a way that supports health.

RELATIONSHIP BETWEEN FOOD AND THE THREE *GUNAS*

In our discussion of the three qualities of the mind in Chapter One, we briefly mentioned the effect that certain foods have on the predominance of *sattva*, *rajas* and *tamas* in the mind. The following list offers a more detailed explanation of the connection between food and the state of mind.

Sattvic Foods

Foods which have a *sattvic* influence on the mind are light in terms of their digestibility and easily nourish the mind and body. They include fresh foods, milk, *ghee*, fresh fruits, most vegetables, grains (especially white and brown *basmati* rice), whole wheat, oats, split or whole mung *dal* (lentils) and almonds. These foods produce calmness, clarity and creativity in the mind and health and vitality in the body.

Rajasic Foods

Foods which amplify *rajas* in the mind increase the heat and activity level in the body. They include onions, garlic, hot peppers, tomatoes, radishes, chilies, corn, spices, eggs, fish and poultry. These foods make the mind restless, more aggressive and emotional.

Tamasic Foods

Tamasic foods, promote heaviness in the body and include red meat, alcohol, mushrooms, deep-fried and fermented foods, aged foods, like cheese and leftovers. These foods cause mental dullness, confusion and disorientation as well as physical lethargy and sluggishness. They also give a violent slant to the aggressive quality of *rajas*.

THREE ASPECTS OF GASTROINTESTINAL VITALITY

In addition to proper diet, *ahara* emphasizes the role of three components vital to healthy gastrointestinal functioning: *deepan*, the maintenance of strong digestive fire; *pachan*, smooth digestion and assimilation; and *anuloman*, proper elimination of waste materials. When these three operate normally, the body will respond well to almost any appropriate treatment. People fall ill because they have problems in one or more of these areas. Many people consider weak appetite, sluggish digestion or constipation as an unfortunate but minor fact of life. They are not aware that these "small" inconveniences can lead to serious disease over time.

Deepan: Good Appetite

Agni regulates the appetite. A strong appetite, called *deepan*, gives the signal that the digestive system is ready for new food intake. If appetite is consistently variable, weak or excessive, or if we experience abnormal cravings, something is wrong with the digestive *agni*. Our appetite should guide us to eat what we need in suitable quantity and at those times when the body can derive optimum benefit from it. If you're not hungry, don't burden your digestion by eating. Let *agni* regain its strength so it can digest what you have already eaten and neutralize any *ama* which has formed. Some simple solutions exist to regain appetite and rekindle *agni*: Drink ginger tea, avoid solid foods and take only liquids for twelve hours.

Pachan: Good Digestion

Pachan or healthy digestion assures proper nourishment of the *dhatus*. When digestion is impaired, we may experience acidity, gas, bloating and nausea, as well as a sour or metallic taste on the tongue. These things indicate that digestion is sluggish and *ama* is being produced. The body always gives us signals when we have eaten something unsuitable. Most people ignore these signals. If you feel that your digestion is not strong yet you still have some appetite, then eat only a small amount of easily digestible food.

Anuloman: Good Elimination

Improper elimination manifests as irregular bowel movements, consistently loose bowels, constipation, hard or sticky stools. These show that toxins and waste are accumulating and fermenting in the colon, making it pH acidic and disrupting absorption and elimination. If your bowels are not moving, additional food will only increase the burden on an already sluggish colon. Take only liquids or skip a meal to give the body a chance to re-establish normal colon function. Healthy elimination, called *anuloman*, occurs first thing in the morning, so that the system is free to accept the day's new food.

When appetite, digestion and elimination are normal, we have abundant energy, strong bodies, good health and clear minds. Sleep is deep and refreshing. Ayurveda's focus is on the strength of the patient, not the disease and sees illness result from the weakness of the patient. When an individual is strong, resistance to disease is strong.

We cannot avoid the death of the body, but we can do a great deal to prolong life and improve its quality. We can enjoy a long and productive life without medical complications and without the suffering that accompanies debilitating illness. In that light, we offer you the simple cleansing procedures contained in Chapter Twelve that you can do for yourself. They will help minimize or even negate the potential for any future need for medical intervention.

VIHARA: LIFE-SUPPORTING ACTIVITY

The second pillar of *ayu* is *vihara*, or "activity." This principle explains how to act in ways that support life, and includes lifestyle guidelines to maintain optimum health and balance. Successful use of *vihara's* recommendations depends on the ability to know exactly what is good for us and the motivation to act on what we know. This is why a *sattvic* mind is so important. So, many of the following lifestyle suggestions have, as their primary focus, to refine the quality of the mind.

Meditation

The endless number of demands on our time and attention keep our minds constantly active. In addition, the negative influences from our environment create fear and confusion. These influences cause our mind to be confined to a superficial level where it is either too scattered or too dull to experience the vast physical, mental and emotional resources that lay hidden within us. This may explain why scientists estimate that most people use only a small fraction of their mental potential. The limitless possibilities that exist in the subtler levels of awareness remain inaccessible except to a calm, settled mind.

Only when we are strongly influenced by *sattva* do we gain access to those calm, creative and comprehensive levels of awareness that allow us to appreciate the whole of life as well as its parts. There is perhaps not a more effective way to enhance the quality of *sattva* than meditation. That is why the first recommendation of *vihara* is the daily practice of meditation. Throughout history, every great civilization has endorsed regular meditation as a way to enhance all aspects of life. It is a misunderstanding of its purpose to see meditation as an escape from the responsibilities of life, or as a luxury or indulgence. Meditation is, in fact, a necessity, particularly given the fast and stressful pace of modern life.

Meditation allows us to transcend our active phases of the mind and directly experience ourselves as *param atma* in the still, silent, unified quality of mind. Research has shown that meditating significantly restores balance in life and creates dramatic improvements in physiological and psychological health. Meditation causes us to become increasingly sensitive to the needs of our bodies and spontaneously start to make choices which promote health.

Rest

Staying rested is another key aspect of *vihara* which promotes *sattva* in the mind. Fatigue is a major contributor to the mind's loss of "knowingness." Most of us notice how inefficient and dull we become after a night of little sleep — it seems to take an hour to accomplish what we would normally do in ten minutes. This is, unfortunately, all too common an experience since the demands of modern life cause many of us to "burn the candle at both ends." A major key to staying rested is: Go to bed early and wake up early. If we sleep when nature sleeps and wake when nature wakes, we attune our lives to nature's cycles instead of resisting them. So much energy is needlessly expended in resisting the natural cycles of life.

Meditation and rest exist in our nature to create quiet in us. This allows the body and mind to release stress and toxins. You can observe the same phenomenon in nature. For example, during the full moon the ocean is at high tide; it is intense, active and holds everything. During the new moon, the ocean is calm; this is the time, for instance, when garbage washes up onto the shore. This demonstrates how nature removes her wastes during the time of calm and quiet. Similarly, if we allow the mind and body to meditate and take rest, that will release stress and waste materials from the body.

Vihara also advises us to work in moderation. Getting exhausted in the pursuit of our dreams negates our ability to enjoy our achievements. In all cases, desires are more easily fulfilled when they are created from the clear, comprehensive, *sattvic* levels of mind where we have maximum support from nature's infinite organizing intelligence.

Exercise

Vihara prescribes two types of exercise to enhance the quality of our lives. The first is cardiovascular or aerobic exercise, which stimulates muscle metabolism and increases oxygenation. It also strengthens and improves *mamsa* and *meda dhatus*, along with the performance of the heart and circulatory system. This type of exercise should be done frequently, under the advice of your physician. It is essential to take your *vikruti* into account when performing this sort of exercise. *Kapha vikruti*, for instance, generally needs an intense amount of exercise, whereas *pitta vikruti* can handle only a moderate amount. *Vata vikruti* should exercise less than *kapha* or *pitta*, because *vata* becomes easily aggravated by too much activity.

Vyayama, which means gaining energy by exercising, is the second form of exercise recommended by *vihara*. This definition implies that there is a category of exercise that gives energy to the body rather than causing it to expend energy. The three specific forms of *vyayama* are called *surya namaskar* (sun salutation), *yoga asanas*, and *pranayama*. Unlike aerobic exercise, these stretching and breathing exercises are done in a very slow and gentle manner, and serve to lower cardiovascular activity rather than speed it up. After their performance, we actually feel more light, invigorated and clearer than before.

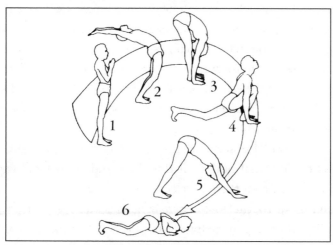

Surya Namaskar — Sun Salutation

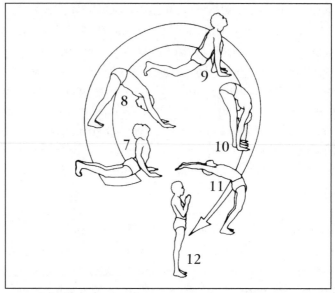

Surya Namaskar — Sun Salutation continued

Why does one feel lighter and more invigorated by *yogasana* and *pranayama* compared to aerobic exercises? To explain this, let me give you a simple example. If you injure your arm or leg, you may not feel very sick. You can heal those injuries without necessarily affecting the rest of your body. However, if you receive an injury to the abdominal area, you can become very ill, resulting in a serious disease manifestation throughout the body. What this shows is that you need to pay more attention to the abdomen rather than to the extremities. That is why Ayurveda suggests *yogasanas* and *pranayama*.

If you carefully observe what *asana* and or *pranayama* do, they exercise the internal organs of the chest and abdominal cavity. Creating pressure on these particular organs helps to remove *ama*, by moving it to the G-I. tract where it can be eliminated. Expanding these organs helps to support the movement of nutrition to the *dhatus*, which insures their proper functioning.

Also, performing alternate nostril breathing exercises help to expand and constrict the chest, diaphragm and hemispheres of the brain. This is a massaging exercise which supports the release of toxins and improves their functioning. This *pranayama* increases the supply of nutrition to all *dhatus* and helps to expel the *malas* from the body. This most important function, performed by the *doshas*, is strongly supported by *yogasanas* and *pranayama*. That is why *Charaka* has mentioned that to use *yoga* along with *Panchakarma* therapy eliminates disease.

In practicing this aspect of Ayurveda (*Panchakarma*), I suggest four important *yogasanas* (postures) to be performed for receiving the complete benefit of this cleansing and rejuvenation program. I recommend these to be used in the daily routine practice (*Dinacharya*): Locust (*Shalabhasana*), Knee-Chest (*Pawan Muktasana*), Cobra (*Bhujangasana*), and *Uddiyan Bandha* (a specific exercise for intestines), in addition to *pranayama* (alternate nostril breathing).

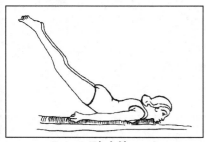

Locust (*Shalabhasana*)

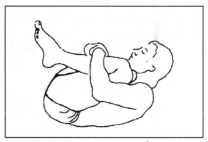

Knee to chest (*Pawanmuktasana*)

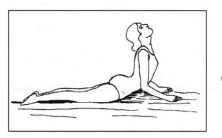

Cobra
(*Bhujangasana*)

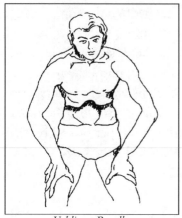

Uddiyan Bandha

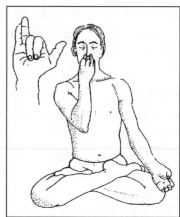

Alternate Nostril Breathing
(*Pranayama*)

You can see that these practices help to release toxins from the abdomen and increase their ability to control digestion and metabolism, while improving *agni* function. So, Ayurveda and *Yoga* give more importance to *Vyayama*, rather than to the build-up of muscles only.

Taken together, these three aspects of *vyayama* provide a number of significant benefits for the body and mind.

They help *vata*'s five aspects or sub-*doshas* to perform their functions properly according to their specific directional orientation.

They accelerate and improve the function of *agni*, which helps maintain a strong, healthy appetite and digestion.

They help maintain the balance of the endocrine system.

They improve and refine sensory functioning.

They release stress, calm the mind and increase *sattva*.

They enhance *rasa* and *rakta* metabolism which improves the circulation of lymph and blood.

To gain maximum value from these exercises, practice them just before meditation and in the following order: (i) sun salutation, (ii) *asanas* and (iii) *pranayama*.

Sensory Experience

We have already stated that what we take in through the senses powerfully influences the mind. Attention moves from the mind out through the senses and the sense organs to the objects of perception and back again. If the objects of attention are either under-stimulating, over-stimulating or toxic, they can disturb the mind's natural equilibrium and directly or indirectly damage the body. Consequently, the senses play a key role in maintaining balance in the mind and body.

The way the senses operate is comparable to eating. If we do not eat enough food, the *dhatus* don't get enough nourishment to perform their functions. If this situation continues, *dhatu* structure and substance diminish and the body becomes emaciated. If we eat too much food, the digestive *agni* gets overtaxed and *ama* forms, again injuring *dhatu* function. Food which is either difficult to digest or poisonous also creates *ama* and ultimately damages the *dhatus*.

Similar processes take place in the mind. When we take in inappropriate sensory stimuli, mental and emotional *ama* form and impair mental functioning. For instance, when we see a violent or horrifying movie, we often have difficulty falling asleep; when we finally do sleep, we're disturbed by violent dreams. As a result, when we wake up in the morning, our bodies feel tired and lethargic and our minds are dull or agitated.

This demonstrates the impact that the senses have on mental and physical equilibrium. The senses are designed to protect us. They relay a vast amount of information to the mind about the body and the environment. Thus, as one of its key components, *vihara* recommends that we use our senses in a life-enhancing manner — a way that supports the mind's ability to make choices which support health and happiness.

Adjusting to Seasonal Changes

We are an integral part of nature. Whatever happens in the environment also takes place in our bodies. We are immediately and intimately affected by changes of season, climate and locale. If our bodies are strong and healthy, we experience these changes as invigorating and revitalizing.

For example, during the cold, damp winter, the elements of *prithvi* and *jala* dominate and *kapha* collects in the body. The body protects itself against the cold by constricting and holding on to its substance. In the spring, when the sun warms the air, the snow melts. Likewise, the accumulated *kapha* liquefies and gets expelled through the dilated *shrotas*. The element of *vayu* becomes lively in the environment, animating the new growth of spring. At the same time, *vata* increases its movement in the body and helps *kapha* eliminate its associated wastes. This "spring cleaning" is the body's way of purifying what is no longer useful so that regeneration and growth can take place.

We can also look at the change that takes place in autumn when summer begins to wane. The winds begin to blow and the leaves dry and fall. *Agni* and *vayu bhutas* now command the environment. The *pitta* which amassed in the body during the summer begins to move out of its normal location when *vata*'s influence grows stronger. People with a *pitta vikruti* suffer from symptoms of excess heat. The body's natural efforts to dispose of toxins and wastes can produce acidity, skin allergies and erratic bowels.

Rutucharya: Seasonal Routine

Though we have given examples of the effects of autumn and spring on the body, each season has its own impact on the balance of the *doshas*. To help each person adjust to the changing influence of the seasons, *vihara* recommends a seasonal-specific, daily routine called *rutucharya*. These simple activities will help keep us healthy throughout the year.

During the spring, mucous secretions become more readily available for elimination. *Rutucharya* therefore recommends *gandush*, or gargling with a warm saline solution, first thing in the morning to clear mucus from the nasal passages and throat. In addition, warm showers dilate the *shrotas*, helping the body expel *kapha*. Continue to dress warmly until the coolness in the environment subsides. In spring, airborne allergens grow abundant. To protect yourself from these irritants, apply *ghee* to the inside of the nasal passages to trap the allergens. *Kapha* gets vitiated during the spring. If it becomes excessive, Ayurveda advises *Panchakarma* therapy with an emphasis on *vamana*.

Agni gains strength in the summer in both the environment and the body. Therefore eat light, easily digestible, more liquid foods, with relatively little spicing. Fruits and juices are good foods for the summer. Reduce exposure to the sun, avoid strenuous exercise and dress lightly. Take a nap during the afternoon to increase *kapha* in the body. *Vata* becomes aggravated in the summer, so follow a *vata*-reducing diet and lifestyle. If symptoms indicate it has become excessive, it will be very useful to undergo *Panchakarma* with an emphasis on *basti karma*.

In the autumn, *vata*'s drying influence increases. Ayurveda therefore recommends the use of internal and external oleation to maintain proper lubrication in the body. As in summer, it's important to increase fluid intake to maintain hydration. Follow a diet which pacifies both *pitta* and *vata* and continue to use fewer spices. Soup and yellow mung *dal* are useful for this. Since *pitta* gets aggravated during the fall, an excess accumulation can be eliminated by undergoing *Panchakarma* with an emphasis on *virechana*.

Cold and dampness reach a peak in winter. Therefore, stay warm, dress warmly, take warm showers and baths and eat warm, spicy food. Continue to emphasize the use of *ghee* and oil internally and externally. During this season, appetite grows as *agni* increases to protect the body from the cold. Increased digestive capacity at this time makes it easier to build up the *dhatus*. *Rasayanas* are therefore recommended during the winter months. *Vata* can manifest excessively during this time. If this occurs, seek out *Panchakarma* therapy with an emphasis on *basti* and *nasya karmas*.

Dinacharya: Daily Routine

In addition to these seasonal guidelines, *vihara* makes recommendations for our daily routine, called *dinacharya*. Anyone can follow this simple set of directions to maximize their health regardless of the season or their particular *vikruti*.

Wake early, preferably at sunrise.

Urinate and defecate upon arising.

Scrape your tongue and brush your teeth.

Drink a glass of warm water.

Perform *abhyanga*, or "oil massage."

Take a warm bath.

Do *asanas* (yoga postures), *pranayama* (alternate nostril breathing) and meditation.

Exercise according to your *prakruti*.

Apply *ghee* or sesame oil to the nostrils before going out.

Do not restrain natural urges such as yawning, sneezing or urinating.

Eat fruit and herbal tea for breakfast. If you feel hungry, eat hot cereal.

Engage in activity that brings you joy.

Eat your main meal at noon in a quiet, settled atmosphere.

Do not overwork.

Reduce rushing, worrying and overeating.

Treat yourself gently and lovingly.

Meditate at the end of your day's activities.

Eat a light meal in the evening.

Go for a walk.

Retire early.

The prescriptions offered by *ahara* and *vihara* are more designed to promote the body's normal, healthy functioning than to rid it of wastes and toxins. Consequently, dietary and behavioral management alone will not cure most well-established diseases. While some diets and activities assist the body's natural detoxification mechanisms and are used as an adjunct during cleansing therapies, once toxins are deeply rooted in the *dhatus*, we must resort to the *aushadhi*, the third pillar of *ayu*. The theme of this next section of the book is the Ayurvedic treatment of disease. The discussion will begin with the nature and origin of the disease process and the procedures Ayurvedic science employs to eliminate the disease at its source. I trust that you will find this second half of the book as fascinating as the first.

Ayurvedic Treatment Of Disease

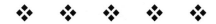

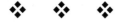

Chapter Seven

THE DISEASE PROCESS

yurveda's knowledge of the disease process differs fundamentally from the conceptions held by Western medicine. Though Ayurvedic science recognizes the role played by viruses and bacteria in disease, it explains that these pathogens cannot cause illness by themselves. Both our bodies and our environment harbor vast numbers of the microorganisms which modern medicine believes to be the source of illness. What actually determines which person will succumb to the influence of these pathogens and which will remain healthy? What are the unseen factors involved in the creation of illness?

There are many modern treatments that effectively destroy the microorganisms which cause many diseases, but in a high percentage of cases — venereal diseases and tuberculosis, for example — symptoms recur after a few years. Anti-bacterial and anti-viral therapies may work in the short term, but they do not seem to eliminate the weakness and susceptibility which allow these diseases to reappear. Such evidence indicates that the allopathic view of pathogenesis is incomplete. To locate the origin of disease, we must look beyond purely physical factors.

The Three Causes of Disease

Just as we are much more than our bodies, morbidity is far more than just a physical phenomenon. As we explained in Chapter One, Ayurveda's conception of human life comprises four basic aspects: soul, mind, senses and body. All four of these components participate in the creation of health and happiness, and all four play a role in the generation of disease as well. However, Ayurveda sees the mind as the key factor in supporting the vitality of each part of life and maintaining its connection to life's underlying wholeness. The mind ultimately determines the strength or weakness of the body and its resistance or susceptibility to factors which produce sickness.

Definition of Three Causes of Disease

Pragya Aparadha	Mistake of Intellect
Asatymya-Indriyartha-Samyog	Missuse of Senses
Parinam	Effect of Seasons

Pragya Aparadha: The Mistake of the Intellect

Though Ayurveda recognizes three causes of disease, it lists the most important as *pragya aparadha*, "the mistake of the intellect." The intellect makes its most serious error when it identifies with individual objects, or parts of knowledge, rather than the unbounded wholeness which is its true nature. Another way of saying this is that we become identified with our limitations, rather than with our unlimited potential. This situation is extremely stressful for body and mind, since it represents a fundamentally false relationship to life. Most people do not make this choice consciously. The behavior patterns and belief systems inherent in our education and culture precipitate and reinforce the intellect's loss of intimacy with its source in pure consciousness, or knowingness.

Pragya apradha begins at an early age and corresponds with the gradual loss of the mind's *sattva*, its brilliance, innocence and joy. As the influence of *sattva* diminishes, that clear discriminative intelligence within us also starts to fade, and we make other mistakes of the intellect. These errors involve choices in behavior and eating which do not support the natural balance between the *doshas* in our bodies and the elemental principles that govern our environment. Such decisions inevitably create disharmony with the laws that govern nature's functioning, and are, in essence, crimes against our own well-being. When we create disharmony or imbalance in our relationship with nature, we simultaneously create internal disharmony, with disease being the natural consequence.

When the intellect ceases to identify with wholeness, the mind becomes weak and makes choices that injure life and generate illness. For example, take the use of alcohol and cigarettes. All cigarette packaging contains a clear warning about their damaging effects on health. Most people are aware that alcohol and tobacco weaken the immune system and cause a variety of serious illnesses. In spite of all this, many individuals continue to use these things to their great detriment.

Asatmya-Indriyartha-Samyog: The Misuse of the Senses

When the mind loses its *sattva*, it loses its ability to spontaneously make life-supporting decisions, and we begin to use the senses in harmful ways. Ayurveda calls this improper use of the senses, *asatmya-indriyartha-samyog*, and considers it to be the second cause of disease. Chapter One has already explained the three ways that the senses can be misused, namely overuse, underuse or emotionally harmful use. Sensory abuse disables their functional and protective capacity and, consequently, permits harmful influences to impact the mind and body. *Sattva*'s influence in the mind then wanes even more, resulting in *doshic* imbalance and the production of *ama*.

Parinam: The Negative Impact of the Seasons

Once created, *ama* interferes with the *doshas'* ability to maintain a balanced relationship with one another and to operate effectively. Eventually, the *doshas* lose their natural adaptability, preventing them from adjusting to changes in climate or season. They can no longer counter the demands placed on the body by changes in the proportion of *bhutas* in the environment. As a result, more *ama* forms and new seeds of disease are sown. Ayurveda calls the inability to adapt to changing seasons *parinam*, which means "the effect of the elements on the body," and designates it as the third cause of disease.

Though *pragya aparadha* is the ultimate cause of disease, all three of the above factors generate discord between the *bhutas* governing the physiology of nature and the *doshas* governing our individual physiology. When the rhythms of individual life do not align with the cycles of nature, stress, weak digestion and *doshic* imbalances inevitably result.

Once imbalance in *doshic* functioning occurs, pressure is put upon the primary *agni* in the digestive tract as well as the *agnis* in each of the *dhatus*. Debilitated digestive fire impairs the system's ability to efficiently convert food into nutrients. This results in *ama* formation and inadequate or defective nutrition reaching the *dhatus*. When the *dhatus* become toxic and malnourished, immunity breaks down, and pathogens such as viruses and bacteria increase in the body, setting the stage for a host of infectious illnesses and degenerative disorders. From the Ayurvedic perspective, pathogens are, at most, a secondary cause of sickness. In almost all cases, disease on a physical level results first from a breakdown in function, followed by the development of abnormalities in substance and structure.

Shat Kriya Kal: Six Stages Of Disease Manifestation

Modern medicine recognizes two stages in disease formation. The first is the stage of detection, where clearly distinguishable symptoms have begun to manifest. Complication is the second stage, where disease is so advanced that it effects other areas of the body and is basically irreversible.

Ayurveda, however, elaborates a six-stage process of disease manifestation, called *shat kriya kal*, in which detection and complication comprise the last two phases. Knowledge of the first four stages is unique to Ayurveda and permits the recognition and elimination of disease long before it progresses into clearly differentiated clinical symptoms. *Ama's* toxicity and the *doshas'* mobility (*dosha gati*) constitute the key components in the disease process. We'll now analyze the six-stage development of disease from the point of view of these two factors.

Sanchaya: The Stage of Accumulation

The first phase of disease formation is called *sanchaya*, meaning "stored." It can be understood as the period of accumulation. At this time, *ama*, produced during improper *prapaka* digestion, collects in the gastrointestinal tract. This condition is primarily associated with weak digestive *agni* and an excess in one of the *doshas*. *Ama* associated with a *kapha* imbalance accumulates in the stomach. When *ama* results from a *pitta* imbalance, it collects in the small intestine; and when connected to a *vata* dysfunction, it amasses in the colon. *Ama's* presence disturbs the *doshas'* functions, and creates mild symptoms which the individual can usually feel. We seldom act on these symptoms because they generally disappear by themselves in a few hours.

These symptoms signal physiological imbalance, and when we ignore or suppress them instead of recognizing and eliminating their causes, we invite the disease process to gain a foothold in our bodies. For example, suppose we go out to dinner with friends and drink or eat foods which are difficult to digest. Perhaps we eat too late at night when digestive *agni* is not strong. That night indigestion disrupts our sleep. In the morning we feel heavy, lethargic and maybe even nauseous. Incompletely digested food sits in the stomach and nausea tells us the body wants to eliminate it. At this time we should fast and allow the digestive fire to rekindle so that the food remaining in the stomach can be fully metabolized. Instead, we drink coffee and take an antacid or some other over-the-counter medicine to mask the symptoms and make us feel better.

These symptoms alert us to an imbalance. If not properly addressed, the undigested food and toxic by-products of *doshic* malfunction stay in the body and move into the intestines. By the afternoon, the nausea is gone, but has been replaced by acidity, bloating or some unpleasant or sour taste in the mouth. This happens because the undigested food has now moved into the *pitta* zone. We may take another antacid or eat again, even though we don't feel very hungry, further burdening the digestive fire. Our energy is low, but by the evening or the next morning, we start to feel better again.

Once the nausea, acidity and bloating disappear, we have missed an opportunity offered by the body to eliminate the cause of future disease. The symptoms do not leave because we are better, but because *ama* no longer burdens the digestive tract. Although we feel better, our body has started to sow the seeds of sickness.

Prakopa: The Stage of Aggravation

Prakopa, the second stage of the disease process, translates as "aggravation" or "provocation." Once we feel better, we are not inclined to change those aspects of diet or lifestyle which brought the initial discomfort. As a result of not heeding the warnings arising from our digestive discomfort, we continue to make the same mistakes and *ama* continues to be produced. Eventually, *ama* amasses to such a degree that it begins to get active or provoked in the site of its production in the G-I tract, leading to the third phase of disease.

Though the *prakopa* phase does not manifest the clearly differentiated clinical symptoms which allopathic medicine can recognize, the Ayurvedic physician can confirm *ama's* aggravated state through pulse diagnosis. He can then make dietary and behavioral recommendations to reverse the *prakopa* stage.

Prasara: The Stage of Migration

The third phase of disease formation, is referred to as *prasara*, which literally means "to leave and spread." *Ama* accumulates to such a degree that it begins to overflow its site of origin in the G-I tract. Since it can no longer be contained here, the *doshas* transport it, along with essential nutrients, to the *dhatus* by virtue of *dosha gati*, the twice daily movement of the *doshas* from the body's hollow structures to the deeper structures and back again.

The question then arises, if *ama* is carried to the *dhatus*, why isn't it carried back again? The answer has to do with the sticky quality of *ama*. Once it lodges in the *dhatus*, its stickiness prevents it from being transported back to the G-I tract. The migration of *ama* from its site of origin occurs in the same sequence as *dhatu* development: First it is transported to *rasa dhatu*, then to *rakta*, *mamsa*, *meda* and on into the deeper *dhatus*.

Sthana Samshraya: The Stage of Disease Augmentation

Sthana samshraya, or "taking shelter in a place," comprises stage four. The *ama* which has migrated enters and lodges in a weak or defective *dhatu*. Once *ama* accumulates in an area of low immunity, its qualities overwhelm the *dhatu* and cause dysfunction and structural damage. This is the stage in which specific degenerative diseases and susceptibility to serious infection begin. A number of factors determine which *dhatus* are predisposed to accept and be damaged by *ama*: congenital influences; effects from past diet and behavioral choices; effects from previous illnesses, stress, seasonal changes, chemical pollutants and radiation. Often a combination of these factors produces the weakness that opens certain tissues to disease.

Vyakta: Stage of Symptom Manifestation

Vyakta, or "that which can be seen," is the fifth stage, and the one in which clearly differentiated symptoms first appear. The disease process overwhelms the body's ability to maintain immunity and healthy functioning. Structural damage and dysfunction have progressed to the point where the illness activates. Here the disease process manifests the symptoms used by the Western system for classification and diagnosis. Because modern medicine does not have an accurate or complete understanding of the origin of the disorder, its treatments often aim at suppressing or eliminating symptoms without removing their underlying causes. Even when symptomatic palliation is successful, sooner or later the specific disease process will recur or find another avenue to manifest in the body.

Bheda: Stage of Complications

The sixth and final phase of the disease process is called *bheda*, which means "differentiation." Whereas stage five confirms general diagnosis, stage six confirms differential diagnosis. It offers such a detailed understanding of the group of symptoms which have surfaced, that all doubts about the nature of the disease are eliminated. This phase is characterized by severe impairment of *dhatu* function, serious damage to the *shrotas* — the vessels within each *dhatu* — and, often, complications involving related *dhatus*. The disease process can be aggravated by the toxic side-effects of many of the drugs that are used to treat it. At this stage, many diseases become difficult to cure completely.

The consequences of a typical, Western teenager's diet provide a perfect example of the six phases of disease development. Cars, sports, TV and learning about the opposite sex captivate the attention of many adolescents. Diet is not a major concern, particularly a healthy diet. Lunch might consist of pizza and a soft drink, finished off with a candy bar or a chocolate sundae. These heavy, *kaphic* foods weaken the digestive fire and overwhelm the actions of the other *doshas*.

Afterwards, the teenager might experience some slight discomfort, indigestion or acidity, but later in the day he feels better. Perhaps he repeats this experience once or twice a week. Being young and healthy, he doesn't give it a second thought. Teenagers tend to have a sense of invincibility; they believe that no matter what they put into their bodies, they will continue to grow healthy and vigorous. To a certain degree they are right. *Pitta* is now starting to dominate the body at this stage of life and *pitta* governs strength and resiliency.

Little by little, the *ama* that is burdening the teenager's G-I tract gets unloaded onto the tissues of the body. As he grows into adulthood, the accumulating *ama* begins to settle in weaker parts of his physiology. Though no definite symptoms have yet appeared, the body's vulnerable places begin to feel the strain and deterioration caused by *ama*, and for the first time, he senses some loss in vigor, strength and flexibility.

Several years down the line, he wakes up one morning to find that his knees or knuckles are a little swollen and painful. He can still ignore these symptoms and for a while they may go away.

Then one day the pain and swelling begins to interfere with his life to such an extent that he consults a doctor, and finds that he has arthritis. The disease process has reached the later stages. His doctor tells him that he can give him something to reduce the pain and swelling, but he will have to learn to live with the disease.

In reality, he has been living with the illness for a long time. Degenerative conditions and susceptibility to infectious diseases do not develop overnight. It often takes many years, or even decades, of sowing the seeds of dysfunction through inappropriate diet and lifestyle before disease symptoms show up. With proper knowledge of the foods and behaviors which are most appropriate for his particular *doshic* constitution, disease could have been prevented. Prevention is always easier than treatment.

It is, therefore, imperative that our educational system begin to teach children a preventative approach to health. They should be trained to recognize and understand what is taking place in their bodies and make the necessary adjustments.

Now that we have the knowledge of how illness originates and how it manifests step-by-step, in the body, let's turn our attention to the procedures that Ayurveda uses to remove both the symptoms and causes of disease.

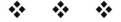

Chapter Eight

PANCHAKARMA: AYURVEDIC DISEASE MANAGEMENT

*A*yurveda uses two main modalities in the treatment of disease, each with its own distinct purpose. *Shamana* therapy is used to palliate or manage the symptoms of disease, whereas *shodhana* therapy is used to eliminate the cause of disease. Each type of disease management has its own appropriateness depending on the patient, the time and the nature and stage of the illness.

SHAMANA CHIKITSA:
Procedures for Alleviating the Symptoms

Shamana, which means "to suppress," reduces or eliminates symptoms. *Shamana* treatments make the patient feel better by suppressing the effects of the body's accumulated *ama*. When we take aspirin to alleviate headache or muscular pain, we are employing a *shamana* or palliative type of treatment. However, *shamana* does not deal directly with root causes of the illness, and thus can never effect a complete cure. Its treatment methods can be compared to cutting weeds off at ground level. While the garden may temporarily appear to be free of weeds, they will inevitably grow back. Similarly, if we do not eliminate *ama*, the source of disease, and change the diet and behavior that created it, the symptoms will continue to manifest.

A childhood experience from my own life illustrates *shamana* therapy. When I was a small boy, I suffered from a case of persistent boils. My mother took me to a dermatologist, who gave me various treatments which eventually caused the boils to disappear. However, it wasn't long before the boils returned as severely as ever.

Fortunately, at about this same time, my grandmother came to visit, bringing with her some valuable folk wisdom. She could not help but notice my condition and asked whether I was constipated. My mother quickly replied that I was lazy about going to the bathroom. Immediately my grandmother gave me a common herbal preparation called *triphala* in a dose large enough to act as a purgative. Within twenty-four hours, my boils were gone. From that point on, my mother saw to it that regularity became a well-established habit first thing every morning and the boils never returned. My grandmother explained to my family that I did not have a skin problem, but was suffering from the effects of constipation. Waste matter and toxins had accumulated in my colon and were being absorbed into my body, thus producing the boils.

At the time, I could not comprehend how taking a purgative could cause skin problems to disappear, and I did not understand the significance of this event until many years later. Shortly after I began my clinical practice as an Ayurvedic physician, a patient came to see me with a serious skin problem. He told me that he had been suffering from boils for a long time and had noticed that whenever he took castor oil as a purgative, the boils went away for awhile. However, they always came back. I then remembered the incident from my own childhood and found the explanation in my Ayurvedic training.

The boils resulted from the body's attempt to eliminate toxins through the skin. As long as the underlying problem was not addressed and *ama* remained in the *dhatus*, the body continued to try to expel the toxins with the boils emerging as a result.

When I was a small boy, one purgation, along with the establishment of regular bowel habits, was enough to cure my skin problems. However, for a thirty or forty-year-old adult, with many years of poor diet, weak digestion and incomplete elimination, purgation alone is not enough to rid the tissues of all the accumulated toxic material. My patient's natural, homeostatic mechanisms persistently worked to help him regain optimum health. Each time the burden on the *dhatus* became too much, the body automatically attempted to bring the *ama* to the surface and expel it through the skin.

Purgation's effectiveness as a symptomatic treatment demonstrated the connection between the mucous membranes of the digestive tract and the skin. The patient's use of castor oil provides a good example of *shamana*, because it reduced the symptoms but did not remove the basis of the dysfunction.

SHODHANA CHIKITSA:
Procedures for Eradicating Disease

The second means that Ayurveda uses to treat illness is called *shodhana*, which literally means "to go away." In this form of treatment, the basis of the disease process is eradicated. *Shodhana* therapy rids the body of *ama* and *mala* and restores balance to the *doshas*. It pulls the weeds out by the roots. It is considered superior to *shamana* because it not only removes the symptoms of disease but also eliminates their cause.

PANCHAKARMA: REJUVENATION THERAPY

All disease processes point to a crisis of *ama* toxicity in the body. *Panchakarma* constitutes the foremost *shodhana chikitsa*, or purification therapy, because it reverses the disease mechanisms which carry toxic waste products from the digestive tract into the tissues of the body.

Panchakarma inverts the movement of *ama*, which takes place in the third and fourth stages of the disease process. During *prasara*, the third stage of disease manifestation, *ama* overruns the site of its initial accumulation in the G-I tract and flows into other areas of the body. During *sthana samshraya*, the fourth stage, the spreading *ama* enters and lodges in weak or defective *dhatus*, where its disruptive influence will eventually produce the final stages of the disease process. *Panchakarma* is designed to draw *ama* out of the *dhatus*, return it to the digestive tract and expel it from the body.

In the case of the man with skin problems mentioned above, when he underwent *Panchakarma* therapy, the cause of his recurring skin eruptions was permanently removed.

The uniqueness of *Panchakarma* is that it puts the attention on the patient, whereas all other therapies focus on the pathology and its symptoms. *Panchakarma* therapy recognizes and uses the specific qualities of the patient's physiological make-up to heal. It does not just treat diseased organs and tissues; it treats and manages the *doshas*, the biological forces which carry *ama* back and forth between the digestive tract and the deeper body tissues.

There is a simple elegance to the approach and effectiveness of *Panchakarma* as a *shodhana* therapy. It takes advantage of the naturally occurring cycles of *doshic* migration, and utilizes the active phases of each *dosha* to draw *dosha*-specific *ama* out of the *dhatus* and eliminate it from the body. In this way, *Panchakarma* differs from every other form of treatment, including all other modes of detoxification and purification.

The name *Panchakarma* comes from two Sanskrit words: *panch*, meaning "five," and *karma* meaning "action." The name incorporates the core of the treatment: the five primary actions or procedures which Ayurveda uses to purify the body of everything foreign to it. Each procedure addresses a specific *doshic* imbalance and the *ama* which forms as a result.

Panchakarma therapy, however, is more than just these five purificatory and rejuvenative procedures. It is a three stage process in which the five core treatments serve as the focal point. The first phase, called *Purvakarma*, comprises essential preliminary procedures whose purpose is to prepare the body to unload stored toxins — the purpose of the main or second stage. The last stage, called *Paschatkarma*, occurs after the main purification processes. It employs a set of procedures to assure the restoration of strong digestive *agni* and thorough rejuvenation of the *dhatus*. These post-procedures are designed to nourish, strengthen and balance the newly cleansed *dhatus*. They aim to establish a consistently healthy energy level, strengthen the immune system and rebuild the body.

To understand how these procedures achieve such a complete physiological purification, we must have a working knowledge of how the *doshas* move in the body. Although we briefly discussed this process in Chapter Three, a more detailed analysis will be beneficial.

Dosha Gati in *Shodhana* Therapy

The *doshas* provide the vital connection between the gastrointestinal tract and the *dhatus*, or deep internal structures of the body. It is important to remember that the *dhatus* comprise the dense, solid structures which do not leave the body, while the *malas* are the natural waste products of metabolism which are removed from their site of origin and expelled from the body.

In the case of the *doshas*, however, they are neither retained nor eliminated and have the unique ability to travel throughout the body. Fluids and semi-solid matter are constantly carried back and forth between the body's hollow structures and its deeper, denser structures through the regular and predictable activity of the *doshas*. They transport nutritive substances from the gastrointestinal tract to the tissues and organs, and also carry unsuitable or damaging substances away from the *dhatus* and back to the gastrointestinal tract for elimination.

A couple of examples demonstrate the widespread effects of this back and forth movement. When we talk a lot, we get thirsty. The movement of air through the mouth exhausts *kapha*'s watery secretions there and the mouth becomes dry. If we stop talking but don't replenish the moisture by drinking water, the mouth eventually becomes moist again. This is because *vata dosha* brings *kapha* from the deeper *dhatus* of the body into the mouth's hollow structure, where it is needed to soothe and moisturize the mouth.

When we exert ourselves in strenuous activity, we get thirsty and our mouth feels dry. Why? Because the *doshas* draw the fluids which are normally in the mouth and digestive tract to *mamsa dhatu* to give extra moisture and lubrication to the muscles. When we drink a lot of liquids during physical activity, we generally do not urinate frequently because the *doshas* are constantly moving the fluids from the hollow gastrointestinal tract to the *dhatus* where they are needed. However, if we drink the same amount of liquid when we are not exerting ourselves, we have a need to urinate more frequently. This is because the denser tissues have no need for the fluid, so the *doshas* remove whatever is excessive and carry it back into the hollow structure of the bladder to be discharged.

In each of these examples, the *doshas* are the components that flow back and forth, transporting fluid between the gastrointestinal tract and the *dhatus*. The *dhatus* can't perform this function because they don't leave their own sites or their own *shrotas*. The *malas* are also incapable of fluid transport because, when they leave their site of origin, they are expelled from the body. The *doshas* constitute the functional intelligences which maintain the body's equilibrium, and sustain it by taking nutrition to the *dhatus* and taking away the *malas*.

As was mentioned previously, when *ama* overflows its site of origin, *dosha gati* moves the *ama*, along with nutrients, to the *dhatus*, where it lodges and eventually manifests as acute or chronic disease symptoms. The *doshas* have the capacity to convey *ama* to the tissues as well as conduct it out of the tissues for disposal. The *doshas* have intelligence. Each of them collects its own type of *ama* and *mala* and brings it to its respective seat in the G-I tract for elimination at a specific time.

Each *dosha* dominates the body twice in every twenty-four hour cycle, in perfect coordination with the *bhutas'* cycle of dominance in the environment. The early morning, when *kapha's* influence takes over, provides the best time to remove *kapha*-associated *ama* from the body. This is when *kapha* naturally moves from the deeper tissues to the hollow structures of the nose and throat, making these watery secretions readily available for disposal. *Kapha* secretions also rise from six to ten in the evening. However, because we tend to be more active at this time, the fluids are drawn away from the G-I tract to the periphery to support the activities of the *dhatus*.

Panchakarmas Related to *Dosha*-Specific Impurities

Vaman Karma *Nasya Karma*	*Kapha Dosha* Zone
Virechan Karma *Raktamokshana Karma*	*Pitta Dosha* Zone
Basti Karma (*Anuwasan and Nirooha*)	*Vata Dosha* Zone

Panchakarma uses two main procedures to remove excess *kapha* and *kapha*-related *ama* from the body. *Nasya*, the inhalation of medicated substances, eliminates toxic congestion in the perinasal sinuses. *Vamana*, therapeutic emesis (vomiting), removes toxic congestion from the stomach. *Panchakarma* generally employs these treatments early in the morning when excess *kapha* is most available in the G-I tract for elimination.

During the *pitta* period (10 A.M. to 12 noon), the processes of digestion, transformation and assimilation are at their peak. Symptoms of abnormal *pitta* function become most evident during this time. The same influences are at work in the two hours before and after midnight. These are the times when *pitta*'s natural movement from the thicker tissues to the hollow structure of the small intestine can most easily assist the removal of *pitta*-associated *ama*. *Panchakarma* then uses the procedure of *virechana*, or purgation, during these times to remove this toxicity from the intestines.

Late in the afternoon, from about 3 P.M. to sunset, *vata* takes precedence and generates more activity in the body. We feel the same effect just before sunrise, when nature, under the influence of *vayu bhuta*, begins to wake up. *Panchakarma* uses *basti* therapy to pacify hyperactive *vata* and eliminate the toxins associated with abnormal *vata* function. *Bastis*, the introduction of medicated and cleansing substances through the rectum into the colon, are more effective when administered in the late afternoon.

Each *dosha* depends on *vata* for movement. We see this everywhere in nature. *Jala* does not contain any inherent impulse for motion. A river, for instance, flows only with the help of *vayu*. The same is true for *agni*. It is *vayu* that causes the flames of fire to leap and dance. Because *vata dosha* initiates and drives all physiological movement, it is considered by Ayurveda to be the master player in all the body's processes. For this reason, *Panchakarma* makes normalization of *vata*'s functioning a primary objective.

Now that we have some theoretical understanding of why *Panchakarma* works as a *shodhana* or cleansing therapy, we can now explore in practical detail, the three stages of *Panchakarma* therapy beginning in the next chapter with the pre-procedures of *Purvakarma*.

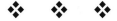

Chapter Nine

PURVAKARMA: PREPARING FOR PANCHAKARMA

anchakarma's five main procedures are designed to eliminate *ama* and restore health to the *dhatus*, but they can only achieve this goal if the body is ready to let go of the accumulated toxins stored deep within its structures. Without proper preparation, these treatments would remove only the *ama* available in the gastrointestinal tract and would have little or no impact on the *ama* lodged in the *dhatus*.

The man whose boils disappeared after purgation, only to see them recur, offers a case in point. The castor oil removed only the *pitta*-associated *ama* which had accumulated in the G-I tract. Why wasn't all of it brought out? It has to do with *ama's* heavy and sticky quality. Once it lodges in the deeper structures of the *dhatus*, it's grasp is tenacious. The *shamana* or palliative therapy used by the man was just not capable of addressing this condition. However, *Panchakarma* permanently eliminated the cause of the boils because it was able to remove the accumulated *ama* that had become stuck in his *dhatus*. In addition, it restored his *doshic* function, normalized his digestion and elimination, and dispelled the potential for future diseases related to *pitta* disorders and *ama*.

THE PREPARATORY PROCEDURES OF *PANCHAKARMA*

The set of procedures which Ayurveda prescribes to facilitate the removal of *ama* and toxins from the tissues is collectively called *Purvakarma*. *Purva* means "before" and *karma* means "actions." These treatments help to loosen *ama* and move it out of the deep structures into the G-I tract, where *Panchakarma*'s main therapies can then eliminate it. The two most important processes used to prepare the system for cleansing are *snehana* and *swedana*. *Snehana* and *swedana* are essential to the success of *Panchakarma*'s deep cleansing. In addition to these, *Purvakarma* utilizes several other *dosha*-specific, adjunct therapies.

Proper administration of the preparatory procedures of *snehana* and *swedana* is essential to the success of *Panchakarma* therapy. Without suitable and sufficient oleation and heating of the body, the main procedures of *Panchakarma* will not achieve deep cleansing.

SNEHANA: OLEATION

Snehana, the first step of *Purvakarma*, saturates the body with herbal and medicated oils. The saturation takes two forms: *bahya snehana* or external oleation, where medicated oils are vigorously massaged into the body; and *abyantar snehana* or internal oleation, where medicated oils are ingested. *Snehana* uses four types of oleaginous substances: vegetable oils (*taila*), clarified butter (*ghee*), animal fats (*vasa*) and fat from bone marrow (*majja*). The oils used match the need of the patient.

Sesame oil (*til*) is the primary vegetable oil used for external application. It is sweet, bitter and astringent in taste, warming in action and easily penetrates and nourishes the skin. It soothes and reduces the effects of excess *vata* without aggravating *kapha* and promotes stability and strength. Sesame and all other oils used in *snehana* are prepared with herbal decoctions to enhance their effectiveness for individual patients.

Herbalized *ghee*, or *tikta ghrita*, the main substance used for internal oleation, is made by processing butter to remove all its milk solids, proteins and water and then cooking it with numerous prescribed herbs. By itself, *ghee* has remarkable properties as a nutritive and medicinal substance. Its effect on the body is quite different from that of butter, and research has demonstrated that it does not tend to elevate cholesterol levels. It contains the least saturated fat of any fatty substance. In proper amounts, *ghee* increases the strength of the digestive *agnis*, while decreasing the heat and inflammation due to excess *pitta*. It reduces excess acidity both in the digestive tract and in the tissues, pacifies *vata* and softens and lubricates the tissues and joints.

Ghee's amazing penetrating qualities make it the most effective substance for internal lubrication. It spreads thoroughly, making it easy for all the tissues to absorb. It carries the therapeutic qualities of the other herbal substances without losing its capacity to increase digestive fire and promote secretions.

Snehana also makes use of animal fat (*vasa*) and bone marrow fat (*majja*) for internal oleation. However, these oils are heavy and difficult to digest, and they can produce excess *kapha* and *ama* if a patient's digestive *agni* is weak. Their use is indicated only for specific disorders such as leukemia and several other types of cancer, as well as certain degenerative disease conditions like myopathy.

In general, *snehana* employs substances with the properties of fluidity and oiliness, which can penetrate even the finest tissues of the body and promote secretions. Each of these properties has a specific effect, but in combination they fulfill five important purposes:

(i) They induce the *dhatus* to give up their accumulated toxins.

(ii) They enhance the secretions through which the *doshas* transport *ama* and *malas* to the gastrointestinal tract for elimination.

(iii) They lubricate and protect the *dhatus* from damage while *ama* is being removed.

(iv) They pacify and nourish *vata* through its unctuous qualities.

(v) They remove the obstructions in the *shrotas* or channels.

Repeated applications of oil to the various mucous membranes promote secretions. If we put a drop or two of *ghee* or oil on the tongue, it generates watery secretions and we begin to salivate within a few seconds. *Snehana* stimulates secretions in the *dhatus* which start to liquefy the glutinous *ama* deposited there. Oil dissolves *ama*'s sticky grip on the *dhatus*, reviving each *dhatu*'s metabolism and reopening its *shrotas* or channels. *Ama*'s viscosity also interferes with the *malas*' natural elimination from the *dhatus*. The secretions have the effect of binding the *malas* together so that they can then be transported out of the body.

Oleation also helps prevent physiological wear and tear. All the body's moving parts experience friction, and lubrication protects these parts from jamming or burning out. Oil lubricates and protects the tissues from loosened *ama* while it is being discharged.

Warm, herbal oils exhibit properties (heavy, slow, unctuous) exactly opposite to those of *vata* (light, mobile, quick), and *snehana* helps restore normal *vata* function, which is essential for disposal of all the body's waste products. *Vata* motivates all motion in the body, and when it becomes excessive, it draws the other *doshas* out of balance. Consequently, *vata* pacification naturally helps quell any disturbance in *pitta* and *kapha*. Oleation also reduces the dryness and coldness associated with *vata*. It soothes, nourishes, lubricates and protects the tissues. Finally, oil aids removal of the *ama*-related obstructions in the *shrotas*, which block *vata*'s natural movement and cause its functioning to become aggravated.

We need both internal and external oleation to reach all seven *dhatus*. The *dhatus* consist of the retainable substances and structures between the hollow G-I tract and the skin. Herbal, medicated *ghee* taken internally penetrates the *dhatus* from the G-I tract out toward the skin; herbalized oil applied externally penetrates the *dhatus* from the skin inward.

Once the oil and *ghee* are absorbed, it is important that they are then excreted from the tissues along with the loosened *ama*. *Snehana* always uses herbal oils to insure that they will not be retained by the body. The herbs not only help the oil to dislodge toxic waste products but also encourage the *dhatus* to expel the oil.

This is accomplished by using predominantly bitter herbs in the oleated substances to promote expulsion. This is because of the body's natural response to the bitter substances. Just as our typical reaction to tasting acrid or bitter foods is to spit them out, our tissues respond by rejecting oleated substances which contain bitter herbs. Though there are 53 herbs used in these formulations, some of the herbs commonly used for this purpose include: *guduchi* (Tinospora Cardifolia), *kutki* (Picrorhiza Kurroa), *haritaki* (Terminalia Chebula), *chitrak* (Plumbago Zeylanica) root, licorice and ginger root. The herbs selected depend on the patient's *doshic* constitution and digestive strength, and the type of *ama* to be removed. The herbs used to prepare *ghee* for internal application also help prevent cholesterol from being deposited in the body.

Oil massage and consumption of herbal *ghee* comprise the primary methods *Purvakarma* uses to oleate the body, however, there are several other types of *snehana* that have more specific effects. Oil can be taken with food, placed in the ears or nose, dripped over the forehead, injected into the rectum or put on isolated areas of the body. These and other adjunctive, preparatory therapies are discussed later in the chapter.

Bahya Snehana: External Oleation

The procedure of *bahya snehana* or external oleation employs a specific form of massage to apply the herbalized oil to the skin, but it should not be confused with the typical massage techniques used in the West. This process uses a traditional style of Ayurvedic massage whereby two, trained Ayurvedic massage technicians work on both sides of the patient simultaneously, employing a series of perfectly synchronized, directional strokes on both the front and back of the body.

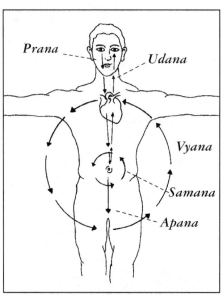

Vata's Five Directional Functions

There is great significance to the strokes used in *bahypa snehana*, for they match the movements of *vata's* five different directional functions. Each function, called a sub-*dosha*, is described below, and has a prescribed *gati* or motion in the body. The specifically designed, directional strokes soothe and nourish the sub-*doshas* and help them take their proper courses.

Prana vayu, the *vata* function which moves from the head, mouth and nostrils to the navel, takes *prana*, or life-force, in the form of air, food and water from the environment into the body. It also controls sensory functioning.

Udana vayu flows in the opposite direction, moving from the navel to the mouth, nostrils and head. *Udana vayu* eliminates carbon dioxide and various forms of *mala*, like mucus and saliva, from the *kapha* zone, and also creates the sounds used in speech. *Udana* originates in the gut, and is the source of our strength.

Samana vayu circulates in a clockwise direction around the navel area. It helps strengthen the digestive *agni* in the same way that air or wind stokes a fire. It is also responsible for keeping the metabolic processes moving in the small intestine and liver.

Vyana vayu moves from the heart to the periphery and from the periphery back to the heart in a circadian rhythm. *Vyana vayu* supports the circulation of the blood and lymph — *rakta* and *rasa dhatu*.

Apana Vayu travels from the navel to the anus and urethra. Its main function is to eliminate urine, feces and menstrual discharge. It is also responsible for childbirth.

Application of *Bahya Snehana*

The Direction of Massage Strokes

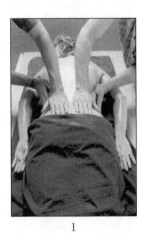

1

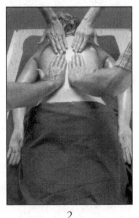

2

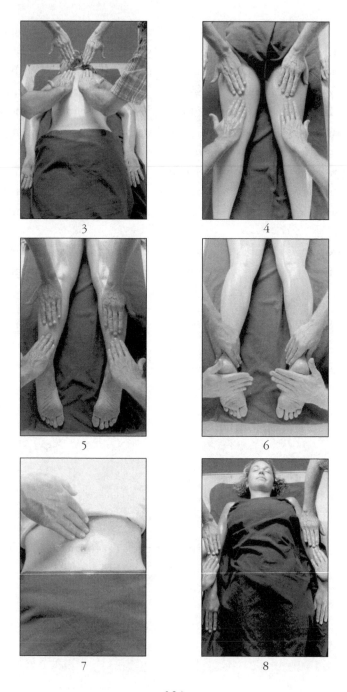

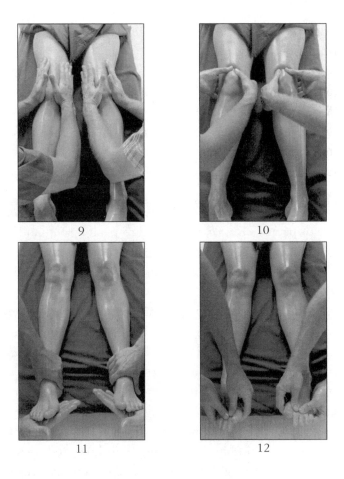

9

10

11

12

Bahya snehana massage progresses through an ordered sequence of strokes, beginning from the umbilius, going to the head, moving back down to the umbilicus, from the umbilicus down to the feet, and from the feet back up to the umbilicus on both the front and back sides of the body.

The pressure of these strokes varies relative to the presence of *marma* points. The *marmas* serve as connecting points between the body's physical substance and its underlying intelligence. *Marma* stimulation enlivens the harmonious coordination among *vata*'s sub-*doshas*, which, in turn, orchestrate every neurophysiological mechanism in the body.

The pressure used during the massage is also geared to push generous amounts of warm, herbal sesame oil into the pores of the skin. We don't often think of the skin as an organ of consumption, but during this process, the skin actually ingests or absorbs a significant amount of oil.

As in so many other aspects of *Panchakarma*, the herbal oils are selected with reference to the patient's *doshic* make-up. Three major types of *dosha*-specific oils are used in *bahya snehana*: *vata shamak*, to pacify *vata*; *chandan bala*, to pacify *pitta*; and *mahanarayana* to pacify *kapha*. Each oil is decocted using the herbs which the *Charaka Samhita* (the main Ayurvedic text) specifies to balance each *dosha*.

Both the massage technique and the herbs allow the oil to penetrate deep into the tissues to loosen the grip of the *ama* lodged there. The *ama* that has formed on the walls of the *dhatus' shrotas* is also loosened, opening up these channels so that *ama* can be more easily removed from the tissues. Though this is the main purpose of *snehana*, it also makes the body supple, increases strength, reduces stress and nourishes the tissues. *Snehana*'s actual meaning implies kindness, tenderness and love, and, true to its meaning, it is a thoroughly soothing and enjoyable experience.

Abhyantar Snehana: Internal Oleation

Abhyantar snehana, or internal oleation, consists of taking prescribed amounts of warm, herbal *ghee*, called *tikta ghrita*, first thing in the morning and in late afternoon on an empty stomach. The Ayurvedic physician gradually increases the prescribed dosage, depending on the strength of the patient's digestive *agni*. The patient does not eat until the *ghee* is digested, which is signaled by the return of appetite.

In preparation for the main eliminative procedures, the patient receives both internal and external oleation each day. These treatments continue for seven days, the time required for the oleaginous substances to reach and saturate all seven *dhatus*. After the seventh day, oleation becomes counterproductive, as there is nowhere else for the oil to go. If continued, it starts to collect in the *dhatus* as saturated fat and depletes the *dhatu agnis*. *Ama* forms, blocks channels and inhibits *vata*'s effective movement. Secondary effects of over-oleating may include poor elimination, hardened fecal matter and abdominal bloating. This is why the major eliminative procedures of *Panchakarma* are always administered after the seventh day of *snehana*.

Certain classical signs indicate oleation's completion. When oil has saturated all seven *dhatus*, the body is well-lubricated, internally and externally. The skin displays a soft and shiny appearance and smells slightly unctuous. Elimination is healthy and fecal matter appears yellowish, shiny or oily, and is softer than normal. Both urine and fecal matter may smell like *ghee*, and the urine may look brighter than usual. Secretions from the eyes, nose and ears shine slightly and the skin and hair become softer. Strength, enthusiasm, energy and clarity of mind all increase.

SWEDANA: THERAPEUTIC HEAT

The second major aspect of the preparatory procedures of *Purvakarma* is called *swedana*, the therapeutic application of heat to the body. Though *swedana* literally means "sweat," the main purpose of *swedana* is not to produce sweat, but to dilate the body's *shrotas* or channels so that oleation's objective — removing *ama* from the *dhatus* — can be more easily achieved. Sweat results naturally when the channels widen. In addition, the application of heat also counteracts the coldness of both *vata* and *kapha*, reduces the body's stiffness and heaviness, and counters the slow, heavy and sticky attributes of *ama*.

As the influence of *agni bhuta* increases, it begins to soften or melt *ama*'s density. *Ama* gets liquefied and shrinks in volume, making it easier to be carried from the tissues. The heating action of *swedana* also mobilizes the *doshas*, which are responsible for transporting these toxic waste materials from the deep tissues to the gastrointestinal tract.

In addition, *swedana* produces tissue expansion, which also facilitates *ama*'s release. Dilating the body's internal channels creates a freer pathway for the removal of toxins and waste products. As *ama* leaves, rigidity and stiffness in the *dhatus* is reduced, giving the body greater flexibility and suppleness.

Primary Types of *Swedana* Used in *Purvakarma*

Swedana assists and enhances the process begun with *snehana*. Many types of *swedana* exist, but the two primary forms used during *Panchakarma*'s preparatory procedures are *nadi* and *bashpa swedana*.

Nadi Swedana:
Penetrating Heat

Nadi, which means "tube," uses steam from an herbal water decoction. In ancient times steam was created in a clay pot and administered to the surface of the body through a bamboo tube. Today, this process is facilitated by the use of a pressure cooker and a nylon

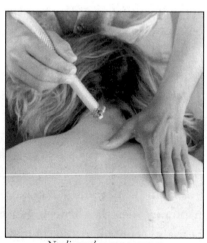

Nadi swedana apparatus

reinforced plastic hose which eases the steam's application to the body's surface. *Nadi* is a more penetrating type of wet heat than *bashpa*, because the steam actively drives the heat and oil (from *bahya snehana*) deep into the tissues through the pores of the skin.

Although this type of steam treatment is given to the whole body, it focuses on the thick and complex structures of the joints to improve their mobility. *Nadi swedana* usually lasts for five to seven minutes. Outside the *Panchakarma* process, it can be used with *snehana* for reducing pain, muscle spasm and rigidity in localized areas. This treatment can be very helpful in the palliative management of backache, inflammation of the spine, hip and knee, and for generalized muscle pain.

Bashpa Swedana: Steam Bath

Bashpa, the second type of *agni swedana*, generally follows immediately after *nadi swedana* is administered. *Bashpa* literally means "steam" and unlike the more directed form of heat used in *nadi swedana*, *bashpa* applies steam evenly to the entire body. *Bashpa swedana* uses a sweat box, in which the patient either sits or lies down on his back. Every part of the body is exposed to the steam except the head, because it cannot tolerate high temperatures. In fact, a technician continuously places cool compresses on the forehead during the treatment to maintain the head's normal temperature. To avoid dehydration, the patient is given a glass of water before administering *bashpa swedana*.

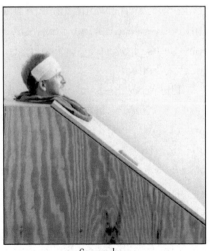

Steam box

191

These small, one-person steam baths are normally constructed of wood with a thermostat that allows their temperature to be easily controlled. Herbal steam is released into the box according to the needs of the patient. The duration of treatment is seven to ten minutes, or until sweat begins to bead on the face and forehead.

The signs of effective and complete *swedana* include sweat, a reddish color to the skin and warmth in the body, with no chill or stiffness. The patient should feel light and more enthusiastic, as the heat liquefies *ama* and its heaviness decreases. It is important not to apply excessive heat, as this aggravates *pitta dosha*. Signs of too much heat include increasingly red skin, faintness, giddiness, exhaustion or feeling burning hot. Breathing difficulty may appear in extreme cases. To counteract theses symptoms and reduce body temperature, the patient can be given cool liquids to drink.

Though *bashpa swedana* is an important preparatory procedure, it is not appropriate for people with heart disease or hypertension, since the heat may cause a rise in heart rate and blood pressure. Individuals with blood disorders, such as anemia or leukemia, also cannot tolerate the temperatures used to induce a full body sweat during *bashpa swedana*. In such cases, *nadi swedana* may be used because its penetrating heat is milder and has only a localized effect.

The procedures of *snehana* and *swedana* are essential to the success of *Panchakarma*'s five main eliminative treatments. The process of purification needs *snehana*'s internal and external oleation to penetrate the deep tissues and liquefy *ama*. It needs *swedana*'s heating effect to dilate the body's channels, mobilize the *doshas* and facilitate *ama*'s extraction and transport back to the gastrointestinal tract.

Without these two procedures, toxins would not be available for complete disposal. If the elimination procedures are attempted without proper preparation, only the most superficial layers of the body are cleansed and the process could place undue stress on the body's tissues. For example, if someone takes a purgative without preparation, it removes only the *ama* in the gastrointestinal tract from the past forty-eight hours. It is similar to trying to squeeze juice from an unripened fruit. The fruit does not produce juice, and is so damaged in the process that it may not be able to ripen and give juice in the future. The preparatory procedures "ripen" or prepare the body in a way that insures that no harm is done to the underlying structures and substances of the body during the cleansing process.

Once the *dhatus* give up their accumulated toxins and wastes and the *doshas* successfully transport them back to the gastrointestinal tract, the body must eliminate these wastes through the closest orifice. This is the job of the second stage of *Panchakarma* therapy.

ADJUNCTIVE PROCEDURES OF *PANCHAKARMA*

A variety of preparatory procedures can be used not only to enhance elimination and purification during *Panchakarma* but to replenish and rejuvenate specific zones of the body. They generally employ some form of *snehana* or *swedana*, and often address the functions of a particular *dosha*. These procedures can also be used outside *Panchakarma*, by themselves, or in conjunction with other treatments, to achieve a specific palliative or nutritive effect either on the whole body or a localized area.

Shirodhara

The most commonly employed adjunctive pre-procedure is called *shirodhara*. *Shiro* means "head" and *dhara* means "the dripping of oil like a thread." This treatment drips warm oil in a steady stream on the forehead, particularly on the brow in the region between the eyes. It is often added to the *Panchakarma* regimen because it pacifies *vata*, in particular *prana vayu*, and calms the central nervous system. It quiets both the mind and the senses which allows the body's natural healing mechanisms to release stress from the nervous system. This, in turn, improves mental clarity and comprehension.

Shirodhara is usually given for twenty minutes, three to four times during a seven-day treatment period. It uses oils made with special herbs that calm and nourish the nervous system and open the *prana shrotas* in the head. The technician administers the oil in a thin stream which flows from a copper vessel hung approximately 6-8 inches above the patient's forehead.

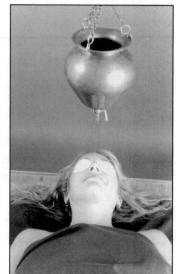

Shirodhara

Pishinchhali

This pre-procedure is popular in South India, where there is a predominance of *vata*-aggravating weather. *Pishin* translates as "squeezing," and *chhali* translates as "vigorous movement." Large quantities of oils are squeezed or poured over the body while massaging it vigorously with a bolus of rice wrapped in a cloth. This drives the oil forcefully through the pores of the skin so it can penetrate into the deep tissues. The treatment is both pleasing and invigorating.

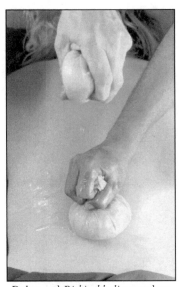
Bolus and *Pishinchhali* procedure

Pishinchhali's most important function is *vata* pacification. It stimulates the *marma* points and creates harmony between *vata*'s five sub-*doshas*. It works in a specific way to eliminate toxins from the joints and improve their mobility. It provides a powerful tool for reducing muscle spasm and degenerative muscle diseases. But in order for it to be truly effective, it must be administered many times in succession. For this reason, *pishinchhali* is often structured as its own separate treatment protocol.

A trained Ayurvedic massage technician administers this treatment for approximately thirty minutes and then follows it with *pinda swedana* (discussed below).

Pinda Swedana

Pinda means "bolus," a soft rounded mass, and *swedana*, as we learned earlier, means "heat." During this procedure, a bolus of hot rice that has been cooked with special *vata*-pacifying herbs is soaked in an herbal milk decoction of nutritive herbs. This hot bolus is then rubbed vigorously over the entire body, focusing on the muscle tissue and joints. It is usually performed after *snehana*, for about ten minutes in most cases, and twenty minutes for more severe conditions.

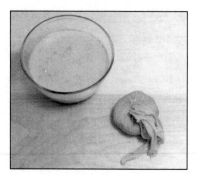

Bolus and milk decoction
for *Pinda Swedana*

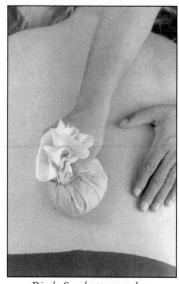

Pinda Swedana procedure

Pinda swedana improves muscle tone and nourishes *mamsa dhatu* and *vata*. It is highly beneficial for treatment of facial paralysis, or hemiplegia, and other degenerative muscle diseases such as multiple sclerosis and muscular atrophy. As with *pishinchhali*, the patient cannot expect to gain results from this procedure with only one or two treatments. Like *pishinchhali*, this therapy is used in conjunction with *Panchakarma*, but for the degenerative diseases just mentioned, it is usually administered as a completely separate treatment program, and performed in a series over a period of time.

Other Types of *Swedana* Used as Adjunct Therapies

There are many methods prescribed by the texts to increase heat in the body, though most are seldom used as a part of *Panchakarma* therapy. Nevertheless, they have a definite benefit and have been employed as effective *swedana* or heat treatments since ancient times. They all involve applying heat directly to the body, generally or locally, and can use heated substances which are liquid or solid, wet or dry, oily or watery, hard or soft.

The Ayurvedic texts describe four main classes of *agni swedana*, each with its own specific purpose:

Tapa swedana, also called *ruksha swedana*, involves the application of dry heat, such as sauna or hot sand fomentation. It is prescribed to reduce inflammation and congestion in the joints.

Upanaha swedana uses hot, herbal poultices prepared with water or oil and may be applied in varying degrees of wetness. The poultices consist of a combination of black gram (*urad dal*) flour cooked with herbs. *Upanaha swedana* is particularly effective in conditions such as gout and arthritis, where the joints are inflamed and painful. The combination of heat, herbs and oil in the poultices reduces pain and restores mobility to the joints.

Drava swedana applies herbal decoctions in hot water, either in the form of a shower or a hot bath. In general, the herbs possess hot, penetrating qualities which enhance the overall heating effect of the treatment.

Ushma swedana uses steam applied either generally to the whole body or locally to the joints and *marma* points. *Nadi* and *bashpa swedanas* described above are the two primary examples of this type of *swedana*. In addition to the benefits already listed, this type of *swedana* has a very beneficial effect on the circulatory system.

LIFESTYLE ADJUSTMENTS DURING *PANCHAKARMA*

Panchakarma is a powerful therapy that provides a unique opportunity for the system to repair and rejuvenate. Those undergoing this program gain the maximum from it if they focus completely on the healing process taking place. That is why an equally important part of *Panchakarma* therapy has to do with the patient's lifestyle during the process. Certain changes in one's diet and daily routine are necessary to insure the greatest results. These lifestyle adjustments begin with the onset of *Purvakarma*, the preparatory phase and continue through the end of *Paschatkarma*, the post-treatment phase.

For *Panchakarma* to work properly, external demands on the mind and body should be removed. The system can then devote its full resources to eliminating toxins and rejuvenating the *dhatus* which have been damaged by impurities. Activity or exertion pulls the action of the *doshas* to the extremities and impairs their ability to transport the impurities from the deep tissues to the G-I tract for elimination.

Ayurveda therefore recommends some lifestyle modifications to maximize the success of treatment, beginning with the onset of the preparatory therapies. Ideally, patients should put aside the usual preoccupation with work and family and devote themselves to rest — mentally and physically. They should have a relaxed schedule and avoid experiences that provoke strong emotions. It's important to forego sexual activity during and immediately after treatment to avoid any undue strain on the body's energy systems. During this time, particularly, patients should not suppress natural urges, such as the need to urinate, defecate or pass gas — the suppression of natural urges always strains the body. Since *Panchakarma* is contraindicated during menstruation, it is important for women to time their treatment schedule accordingly.

Warm, comfortable and pleasant surroundings, free from

drafts, characterize the ideal treatment environment. Baths should always be warm, because the body naturally defends and tightens against cold, whether it's cold wind, water or drinks. Cold influences also decrease *agni*'s effectiveness and impair metabolism. In addition, they shrink the *shrotas* or body channels, which must remain open during *Panchakarma* to permit the flow of *ama* out of the *dhatus* and back to the G-I tract. Through these pathways the healing power of nutrients and medicinal herbs (*rasayanas*) flow to all parts of the body.

During this time it is important to reduce sensory input and give the senses a much needed rest. Because they are the bridge between our external and internal worlds, it gives the mind and body rest as well. Patients are advised to avoid television, bright lights and loud music. If reading is necessary, it is best to do it in moderation. It is also recommended that we minimize speech during the time of treatment. We often don't recognize the effort that goes into producing speech, but it is one of the main ways we expend energy in daily life. Patients should give up strenuous physical exercise during this process. The farther we can pull back into rest, the more dynamic we will be when we spring back into activity once the entire process is complete.

Meditating each day significantly supports successful treatment. Even more benefit comes when meditation is preceded by the gentle stretching and breathing exercises of *asanas* and *pranayama*. The benefit of these things has already been discussed in detail in Chapter Six.

The diet prescribed during treatment by the Ayurvedic physician constitutes a key element in the therapy. If we tax our digestion with heavy food, it interferes with purification and limits the benefits we might otherwise achieve.

The ideal *Panchakarma* diet consists of light, nourishing and easily digestible foods, such as steamed vegetables and *kichari* (yellow mung *dal* and *basmati* rice cooked together with very mild spices). The dietary regimen during *Panchakarma* emphasizes *kichari* for a number of reasons. It does not tax the digestive *agni* and when it enters *prapaka* digestion, it helps to liquefy *ama*. It is highly nourishing, digests easily and calms the mind. Finally, kichari balances all three *doshas*. Here is a good recipe for *kichari*:

Kichari

1 cup split *mung dal* (yellow)
2 cups white basmati rice
1 inch fresh ginger root
1 small handful of cilantro leaves
2 tsp. *ghee* (clarified butter)
1/2 tsp. turmeric
1/2 tsp. coriander powder
1/2 tsp. cumin powder
1/2 tsp. whole cumin seeds
1/2 tsp. mustard seeds
1/4 tsp. mineral salts
1 pinch hing (asafoetida)
8 cups water (6 cups when using pressure cooker)

Wash the rice and *dal* together until the water runs clear. Add the eight cups of water and cook the covered rice and *dal* until it becomes soft. Sauté the mustard seeds, whole cumin seeds, hing, cumin powder, coriander powder and turmeric, together with the *ghee*, in a separate sauce pan and cook for a few minutes. Stir the sautéed spices into the mostly cooked rice and *dal* and cook until done. Add the mineral salts and the cilantro leaves before serving.

The daily diet during treatment should avoid heavy foods which are difficult to digest, such as sweets, fried foods, meat and dairy products. Salty foods, pungent foods (chilies, onions and garlic) and sour foods (pickles, vinegar and citrus) should be greatly reduced. Stay away from fermented foods (yogurt, hard cheese, tofu, soy sauce) and foods with yeast (bread). Ayurveda strongly advises abstaining from cold foods and drinks (ice cream, iced teas and sodas), as well as alcohol and stimulants like caffeine. The *Panchakarma* facility will usually provide the patient with their meals since they know which foods are most conducive to purifying and rejuvenating the body.

If these guidelines are followed from the beginning of the pre-procedures to the end of the post-procedures, *Panchakarma* therapy will be a great success. The patient will enjoy a strong appetite and digestion and feel light and energetic. The mind will be clear and happy and experience satisfaction and enthusiasm for life.

Now that we have explained the primary and adjunctive therapies which Ayurveda uses to prepare the patient for *Panchakarma*, as well as the lifestyle adjustments necessary to insure its success, let's turn our attention to the main eliminative procedures.

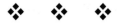

Chapter Ten

PANCHAKARMA'S FIVE
MAIN PROCEDURES

*A*ccording to the *Charaka Samhita*, the body normally uses three routes to eliminate waste products and toxins: the mouth, anus, and pores of the skin. The three *doshas* act as the vehicle which carries *ama* either upward, downward, or out through the periphery. Through *dosha gati*, the *doshas* move these impurities from the deep structures to the G-I tract and from the G-I tract to the body's three main outlets. *Panchakarma*'s curative and rejuvenating power lies in its ability to utilize and stimulate the natural movement of the *doshas* to eliminate *ama*.

Panchakarmas Related to Direction of Elimination of *Ama*

Vamana Karma *Nasya Karma*	Upward Movement *Kapha Dosha* Zone
Virechana Karma	Downward Movement *Pitta Dosha* Zone
Basti Karma	Downward Movement *Vata Dosha* Zone
Raktamokshana Karma	Peripheral Movement Through Blood Vessels

Vamana and *nasya*, two of the five *karmas*, take place in the upper or *kapha* zone of the body and use the upward movement of the *doshas* to remove *ama*. Toxins associated with *kapha* are primarily but not exclusively deposited throughout the upper part of the body. Twice a day, during the *kapha*-dominant periods, *doshic* action draws *kapha*-related toxins into the hollow structure of the stomach from the denser tissues. Because this is where *kaphic ama* naturally collects, *Panchakarma* uses *vamana* or therapeutic vomiting to eliminate them. This is because the mouth offers the easiest and most direct way to discharge these particular types of toxins.

Nasya, or *shirovirechana*, is a procedure used to assist *vamana* in dislodging *ama* and excess *kapha* from the throat, nose, sinuses and other organs in the region of the head and neck. *Nasya* is the introduction of medicated substances into the nose. This process stimulates secretions which help eliminate *kapha*-related toxins from this area. The treatment's primary effect is to improve the connection between the senses and their organs of perception by opening the *shrotas* or channels through which the sensory information flows.

Virechana and *basti* use *pitta* and *vata dosha*'s downward movement to remove related toxins and waste materials from the system. *Virechana* works on the *pitta* zone of the body, whose major organs are the small intestine and liver. *Basti* cleanses the *vata* area, whose focal point is the large intestine. *Ama* associated with *pitta* and *vata* gets discharged from the body through the rectum because of its proximity and accessibility to these organs.

Virechana clears the body and particularly the *pitta* zone of excess *pitta* and *pitta*-related *ama* which naturally accumulates there during the *pitta* times of day. *Basti* therapy introduces medicated substances into the colon through the anus to stimulate the expulsion of *vata*-related *ama* which amasses during the *vata* times. The last of the five major eliminative procedures, *raktamokshana*, removes *pitta*-related toxins from the blood.

These five treatments constitute *Panchakarma's* main purificatory treatments. Let's now examine each of them in greater detail.

Vamana: Therapeutic Emesis

Vamana is one of the least understood of Ayurveda's five elimination therapies. Most people associate emesis or vomiting with nausea and sickness and are repulsed by it. As some of my patient's have said, "Just the thought of vomiting makes me vomit!" However, the emesis procedure used in *vamana* is quite smooth and painless, with little or no nausea, retching or discomfort. This procedure for discharging excess *kapha* and *kaphic ama* was designed to be accomplished with great ease. When the body is properly prepared and the treatment correctly administered, *vamana* is effortless, and effectively removes toxins from the *kapha* zone.

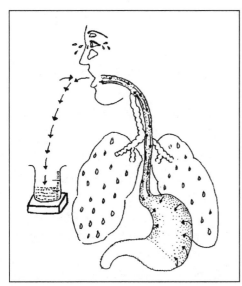

Upper half of body showing emetic action of *Vamana*

The herbs used to produce the emetic effect provide the main keys to successful *vamana*. These herbs, such as *yashti madhu* (licorice) and *madan phal* (Randia Dymotorum) stimulate the action of *agni* and *vayu bhuta*. They are hot, strong and penetrating. Their action permeates the fine channels in the *kapha* zone and stirs up and liquefies the *ama*. Just as fire always

205

moves upward, the heating action of these herbs creates an upward motion which lifts *ama* out of *kapha*'s seat in the stomach.

Vamana is not for everyone. It is usually administered only for *kapha*-related disorders or *ama*. These include: all lung problems, bronchial asthma, allergies, chronic colds, rhinitis, diabetes mellitus (*prameha*), arteriosclerosis, rheumatic diseases, arthritis and some chronic skin disorders like eczema, psoriasis and leukoderma. It is also beneficial for some viral disorders, like Herpes Zoster.

Vamana therapy is contraindicated for people who are emaciated or very weak, the elderly who are frail, young children and pregnant women. People with tuberculosis, pleurisy, collapsed lung, hepatitis, degenerative or cirrhotic diseases of the liver, severe heart disease and problems with blood pressure should also not undertake *vamana* therapy. For these people, as well as those with a severe *vata* imbalance, *vamana* may be too challenging a procedure.

Before describing the specific procedure of *vamana* therapy, I would like to share some experiences in my clinical practice of *vamana*'s effectiveness. A man came to me with a severe skin disorder. He was covered with eruptions, oozing red patches that constantly itched. The doctors he had consulted were baffled by his condition, since it appeared to have some of the characteristics of both eczema and psoriasis. The medicines prescribed for him had a short-term, palliative effect, but the symptoms always returned. He consulted a homeopath whose treatments created some improvement, but after three months, his condition became highly aggravated and could not be controlled by any means.

When he came to my clinic, he was so miserable that he confessed he could not go on any longer. His symptoms indicated to me that he suffered from a crisis of *ama* toxicity. I explained *Panchakarma* to him and took him through the preparatory procedures. After three days of *snehana* and *swedana*, the reddish color of the skin decreased, the itching diminished and the oozing stopped. On the seventh day of the pre-procedures, even before undergoing the primary cleansing treatments, his symptoms had already abated by about eighty-five percent. We were both pleasantly surprised. After completing the *shodhana karmas* and the post-treatment procedures, his skin returned to normal.

Another related situation occurred in the first few years of my practice. A concerned family brought me a twenty-four year old woman with chronic allergic bronchial asthma. She had been taking steroids and using a bronchodilator for many years. Every month or two she would have an attack that required hospitalization in order to manage her symptoms. She had not been able to find anything that would bring her condition under control, and had become depressed and suicidal.

When she arrived for treatment, I found that she had been experiencing poor digestion and elimination since childhood. On my suggestion, she underwent several series of *Panchakarma* treatments, with an emphasis on *vamana*, *nasya* and *basti*. After ten months, her episodes ceased. I began tapering off her use of the steroids and bronchodilator, and after another series of treatments, she was totally free of her dependency on them. She has since married, had a baby and been leading a normal life. She learned to follow a healthy diet and lifestyle, and occasionally takes some herbs to keep her digestive *agni* strong and to ensure the elimination of toxins.

Proper Preparation for *Vamana*

To prepare for *vamana*, *snehana* and *swedana* (oleation and heating) is administered for seven days, after which time the patient should show signs of complete internal and external oleation. In the last chapter, we mentioned that the Ayurvedic physician confirms this by looking for a soft, shiny and slightly oily quality to the patient's skin. He also examines the feces for a similar shiny, oily quality, as well as for increased quantity. When the *dhatus* get fully lubricated, the excess oil and *ghee* become evident through the oily smell emanating from the body and the feces. At this point, the patient is ready and *vamana* can be planned for early the next morning, during the *kapha* period.

The night before *vamana* is administered, the patient takes food which stimulates *kapha* — sweet, heavy, cool, sticky, slimy and oily foods, including yogurt, milk, bananas and *urad dal* (black lentil soup). They increase the volume in the stomach, and this provides the impetus for *kapha*-associated toxins to be expelled, as the stomach cannot hold the increased quantity.

Just before going to bed, the patient is given an herb to stimulate stomach secretions which further increase the volume of its contents. This herb, called *vacha*, has been used by Ayurveda for thousands of years for this purpose. Its energy is hot and causes the *ama* in the stomach to thin out. Because heat rises, *vacha* works in an upward direction, supporting emesis. Patients receive small doses of less than one gram. After taking *vacha*, (Acoromus Calamus) they consume no additional food or liquid until the *vamana* procedure is administered. The patient is advised to refrain from most activity the evening prior to treatment and to retire early since excess activity draws away the *doshic* concentration from the stomach. Meditation always helps produce a calm, settled state of mind and body.

When he awakens, the patient urinates and defecates as usual, but refrains from eating and drinking. An empty stomach stimulates secretions from the surrounding tissues and encourages them to enter the stomach. The patient then receives light *snehana* and *swedana* to increase body temperature and insure that the tissues are expanded and the body's microfine channels are dilated. Most people are unfamiliar with *vamana* therapy, so it is essential that the Ayurvedic physician remain with the patient to provide both technical expertise and support, as well as reassurance. As a word of caution, this is an extremely delicate procedure and should only be performed by an Ayurvedic physician specially trained in *Panchakarma* therapy.

Administration of *Vamana*

Vamana is always given early in the morning, when *jala bhuta* dominates the external environment and *kapha dosha* dominates the body's internal environment. Normal *doshic* activity causes maximum watery and mucous secretions to accumulate in the *kapha* zone during this time, bringing *kaphic* toxins out of the *dhatus* and into the hollow spaces of the stomach. Early morning, when the greatest amount of *kaphic ama* is available for elimination, offers the optimum time for this process.

The procedure begins by giving the patient approximately 300 milliliters (1 1/2 cups) of a thin, sweet-tasting porridge made from wheat and milk. This promotes watery secretions, and again increases the volume of the stomach's contents. The porridge is pleasant and soothing to the taste, and reduces the patient's anxiety about the treatment.

After he eats the porridge, the patient receives an emesis-stimulating herb which contains a strong influence of *agni* and *vayu bhuta*. Such herbs have astringent and bitter tastes which help draw moisture and impurities into the stomach from the surrounding tissues. Classical Ayurvedic texts mention 355 such emetic substances. The fruit of the *madan* tree, called *madan phal*, is commonly used. The fruit's dried powder is soaked in honey overnight and made into a paste. Approximately one-half teaspoon of this pleasant-tasting paste is given to the patient to lick.

To insure that the emesis is as effortless and comfortable as possible, the patient receives a large quantity of warm licorice tea, prepared as a cold infusion the night before. Licorice, or *yashti madhu* (Glycyrrhiza Glabbra), provides an excellent medium for moving sticky, heavy, oily impurities out from the tissues. It belongs to a class of herbs which are not converted into bodily tissue and which stimulate secretions without being absorbed into the tissues. It moves through the body, collecting substances which do not belong to the *dhatus* and is then excreted. Licorice begins building volume rapidly so that the patient suddenly experiences his stomach emptying smoothly, in bouts without retching. If a patient is averse to licorice, sugarcane juice or a saline solution is used.

The patient is asked to drink as much licorice tea as possible during *vamana* to fill the stomach completely (as much as four liters or one gallon). This helps to liquefy the contents, which facilitates their removal. Within a few minutes, the patient feels hot, his stomach churns and he begins to feel the urge to vomit. Salivary secretions fill his mouth and he spontaneously starts vomiting. The patient is encouraged to allow his stomach to empty without resisting. Vomiting comes in bouts and usually occurs smoothly, without strain. A properly prepared patient will not feel sick or uncomfortable. Vomiting is a natural reflex like defecating or sneezing, and the body does not have to exert itself unduly.

Within an hour, the entire procedure is usually finished. The substances used to induce vomiting work for thirty to forty minutes and then their effect naturally subsides. Because of the wheat porridge and licorice tea, the initial taste of the vomitus will be sweet and not unpleasant. The patient should continue vomiting until there is a bitter, sour or burning taste in the mouth. This indicates that the stomach is empty and the contents of the small intestine are now being discharged.

At this point, the urge to vomit automatically stops and the procedure ends. If some of the licorice tea has entered the small intestine, it will come out with the next few bowel movements. The patient should be told that it is not uncommon to have two or three loose bowel movements during the next twelve hours .

When the vomiting stops, the patient should rest and avoid stress as well as any physical or sexual activity for the remainder of the day. He should also abstain from food and liquids for four to five hours, after which time he can take some thin rice water. *Vamana* temporarily exhausts the digestive *agni*, so after treatment the patient needs food which is easily digestible and which will allow the digestive power to rebuild slowly.

Heart rate and blood pressure rise naturally during *vamana*. These should be monitored during the course of the treatment in cases where caution is necessary. The physician measures and compares the amounts of porridge and licorice tea that are ingested, as well as the vomitus that is expelled. A patient may commonly ingest three liters (about three quarts) and vomit out four liters (about four quarts). The difference represents the *ama* and excess *kapha* which have been eliminated from the body. The physician carefully observes the vomitus for color, consistency and odor, which gives him detailed information on the treatment's effectiveness.

Vamana benefits all *kapha* disorders. It leaves the patient feeling light and aware. His senses function with greater clarity and precision. Patients who have suffered with nasal or bronchial congestion notice that their breathing becomes much freer and easier. With proper post-*vamana* follow-up, patients will also find that their digestion is greatly improved.

The body naturally wants to eliminate the toxicity which impairs its functioning, and *vamana* is a natural procedure to eliminate *kapha*-related impurities. With good preparation and administration, *vamana* is as effortless and as easy and spontaneous as yawning or sneezing. It uses the body's innate mechanisms for disposing of damaging substances. As a result, the patient gains immediate relief from the symptoms produced by toxins associated with *kapha*.

Nasya: Therapeutic Cleansing Of The Head Region

Shirovirechana and *nasya* are terms that are used interchangeably. In Sanskrit, *shiro* means "head," and *virechana* means "purging." This procedure purges and rejuvenates the tissues and organs of the head and neck. It introduces medicated oils and powders into the nose, the nearest access and outlet to the organs of the head. It removes *ama* and toxins from the nose, larynx, pharynx, mouth, para-nasal sinuses, ears and eyes. Ayurveda describes the nose as the doorway to the brain. *Nasya* cleanses and opens the channels of the head and improves oxygenation — the flow of *prana* — which has a direct and highly beneficial influence on brain functioning.

Nasya is indicated in diseases of the head and neck. It is used for dry nasal passages, as well as sinus congestion, common cold, chronic sinusitis, allergies and allergic rhinitis. It relieves chronic vascular headaches, migraine, epilepsy, and has a positive effect on degenerative diseases of the brain and mental retardation. *Nasya* also helps with eye and ear problems, such as dry, itching and watery eyes, conjunctivitis, glaucoma, hearing loss and tinnitus, as well as loss of the sense of smell.

The only cases in which *nasya* is contraindicated are for infants who are dehydrated, or for those who are experiencing severe panic or anger. It should also not be administered immediately after bathing. Some caution is advised when giving this therapy to pregnant women. Otherwise, anyone from age eight to eighty can be treated by *nasya*

A classic example of the therapeutic benefits of *nasya* treatment was a man who had been suffering for twenty years with chronic migraine headaches and allergies. He said he had been taking pain medication daily in order to be able to work. During his examination, he mentioned that whenever he felt nauseous and vomited, he felt better. This immediately indicated to me that *kapha*-related *ama* had collected in the region of his head and stomach. I designed a cleansing program for him that began with seven days of *nasya* treatments as well as *snehana* and *swedana*. This had remarkable results. He enthusiastically told me that for the first time in ten or fifteen years, he was waking up in the morning feeling free from pain and heaviness in his head.

His condition improved with this therapy until I felt he was properly prepared for *vamana*, *virechana* and *bastis*. After these treatments, his symptoms were completely gone. The *ama* which blocked normal activity in the *kapha* zone had been dispelled. I have since treated countless patients suffering from long-term, chronic sinus congestion and migraines. In some cases, the conditions had progressed to the point that tinnitus, hearing loss and other complications had developed. The cleansing treatments have, in all cases, produced either a complete cure or a significant improvement.

Another example of *nasya*'s effectiveness is the case of a patient who came to me with clinical symptoms of chronic colds and allergies. He had been suffering from these problems for the last ten to fifteen years. With the onset of the fall or spring seasons, his problem would become aggravated, and make his life miserable. He tried all kinds of therapies, with little benefit. I administered a series of *nasya* treatments over a three week period immediately before the spring and autumn seasons. This cleaned the sinus zones and improved their resistance to infection and allergens. This successfully eliminated his symptoms and dramatically reduced his episodes of colds and allergies.

Types of *Nasyas*

Traditionally, *nasya* uses two different classes of substances: medicated powders and medicated oils. According to *Charaka*, both classes can be utilized for three different purposes:

(i) to promote secretions which dislodge and carry toxins out of the body, called *shodhana nasya*;

(ii) to create a palliative or soothing effect, called *shamana nasya*;

(iii) to provide nourishment to the tissues in the region, called *bruhan nasya*.

According to the needs of the patient, each of these three effects can be increased by varying the substances which are introduced into the nose. *Tikshna shirovirechana* is a *shodhana* type of *nasya* which uses herbs in a sesame oil base. These strong herbs are hot, pungent, dry and quickly penetrating. They increase secretions which help remove *ama* from the nose and head. This treatment effectively eliminates headaches, heaviness in the head, nasal congestion and swollen lymph glands.

Shamana and *bruhan* are palliative and nourishing types of *nasyas*, and generally incorporate sweet materials like *ghee*, sweet herbs (e.g., licorice) or flowers into their formulas. *Shamana*, which means "palliative," helps manage symptoms but does not heal the cause of a condition. For example, when nasal passages are blocked or congested, *vacha* in a sesame oil base rapidly clears the obstruction and returns the patient to easier breathing. This is particularly useful for people with bronchial asthma. *Shamana nasya* helps control sneezing and nose bleeds.

Bruhan, meaning "nutritive," is more nourishing than cleansing. It improves sensory functioning and attention deficit disorders, and helps with degenerative brain conditions like Alzheimer's, epilepsy and mental retardation. The dosage usually begins with eight drops in each nostril and can increase to fifteen drops. *Panchendriya vardhan* oil is commonly used for these conditions. For thousands of years, the herbs in this formula have been known to rejuvenate this area of the body. They include: *Ashwagandha* (Witharia Somniferra), *Pippali* (Piper Longum), *Naga bala* (Sida Cardifolia) and seven other rejuvenative herbs.

Administering *Nasya*

Charaka describes a number of ways to administer *nasya*. The first, *avapidana*, or "squeezing," drips juices extracted from fresh herbs into the nasal passages. This cleanses and soothes the paranasal sinus area. The astringent juices of common grass, for example, can be used to stop a nose bleed. Ayurveda employs *avapidana* for insomnia, headache and anxiety.

The second method for administering *nasya* is *pradhamana*, which translates as "forcefully pushing." It has a strong cleansing action and gives immediate relief from dizziness, fainting, severe headaches and disorientation. In *pradhamana*, powdered herbs are blown into the patient's nose through a tube while the patient inhales deeply.

Marsha nasya and *prati marsha nasya*, or "repeated application," are milder procedures than the previous two *nasyas* because they utilize fewer and weaker herbs and are not propelled as deeply into the nasal passages. Most of the herbs are decocted and applied in a sesame oil base. *Marsha nasya* introduces two to four drops of medicated oil into the nostrils every two hours.

In *prati marsha nasya*, the patient himself applies the medicated oils frequently during the day. He inserts his little finger into warm oil and gently massages the inside of the nasal passages. In both cases, once the oil has been inserted, the head is tilted back and the patient gently sniffs. This treatment cleans, lubricates and strengthens the mucous membranes, keeps the nasal passages open, and increases resistance to foreign substances.

Preparing for *Nasya* Treatment

Proper preparation is crucial to all of *Panchakarma*'s elimination procedures, including *nasya*. Before the medicated drops or powders are administered, warm herbalized oil is vigorously massaged into the face, focusing on the sinus areas. Fomentation, using a hot water bottle wrapped in a hot, moist cloth or towel, is then applied to the face and neck to dilate the passageways. Ayurveda generally prohibits applying heat to the head, but this process provides one of the few exceptions.

Application of *Nasya* Administration

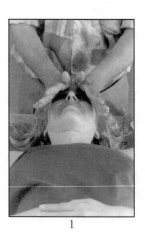 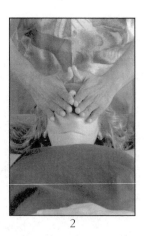

1   2

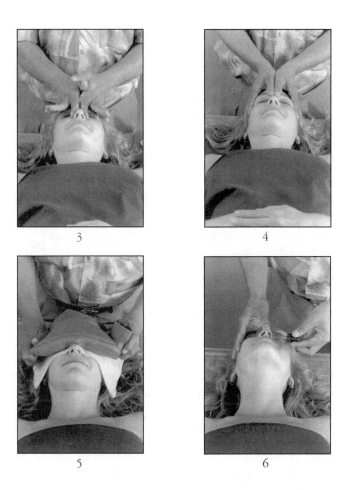

3

4

5

6

After this localized *snehana* and *swedana*, the patient has his head tilted back and receives either herbalized drops in each nostril or powders forcefully blown in. The patient inhales deeply through the nose to bring the herbalized oil up into the sinus passages. To draw the medications more deeply into the passageways, the patient pinches his nostrils closed on the inhale and releases suddenly. He does this quickly, five to ten times per each strong inhale.

If the treatment uses many hot and penetrating substances, we tell the patient that the nose drops may cause a temporary burning sensation. Talking at this time, however, should be kept to a minimum. After a while, the dislodged *ama* and *kapha* begin to flow back into the hollow channels of the mouth, throat and nose. The patient then expectorates or blows his nose to remove these accumulated secretions.

If the patient's nasal passages are inflamed because of excess *pitta*, he may experience burning from the *nasya* treatment. This can be alleviated by placing two drops of *ghee* in each nostril or by placing a cool towel over the face. This eases the dilating and penetrating action of the herbs. After *nasya* the patient rests and avoids exposure to stress, strain or anger.

Treatments start with four drops of herbalized oil in each nostril. As little as one drop is used if the patient is sensitive or if the herbs are particularly strong. Generally, treatment is performed for seven days in a row. After a rest period of a few days, treatment can be repeated for fourteen days and then twenty-one days. A series of treatments of increasing duration may be necessary to treat certain conditions, such as migraine, epilepsy and allergies.

For *kapha* disorders, cleansing *nasya*, using hot penetrating substances in oil, should be applied during *kapha*-dominant periods of the early morning or early evening. *Nasyas* for *pitta* and *vata* conditions are soothing and nourishing. For *pitta* conditions, indicated by nose bleeds and burning sensations, *ghee* is often used and is generally administered at midday or midnight. For *vata* conditions, *nasya* is performed in the late afternoon. As part of the overall *Panchakarma* program, it is best to offer *nasyas* daily, right after *snehana* and *swedana*.

After completing *nasya*, the patient's head will feel lighter and less congested; her mind clear and her senses more acute. She will also feel more comfortable and happy. However, if improper herbs or dosages are used, the patient may experience discomfort. *Nasya* works in the sensitive area of the body close to the brain, and it is vital that it be properly administered.

As we have said, the nose is the gateway to the brain, so it is important to keep the nasal passages and the para-nasal sinuses clear of excess mucus and toxins so that they can function properly. These channels bring *prana* or life-force to the brain and surrounding tissues and protect the body by filtering out potentially dangerous airborne substances or allergens.

VIRECHANA: THERAPEUTIC PURGING

Virechana is a purgative treatment that cleanses the small intestine and associated *pitta*-dominant organs (e.g., the liver and gall bladder) in the mid-zone of the body. It works in a downward direction to eliminate *pitta*-related *ama* and excess *pitta* in the form of acidic secretions. Since *pitta* has a close connection with the blood, it also helps remove waste matter and toxicity from the blood.

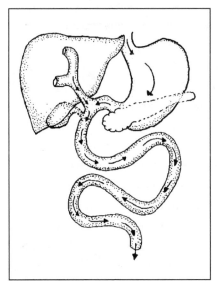

Purging from small intestine through anal orifice

While *virechana* involves the use of strong purgatives which induce loose bowel movements, it affects the body quite differently than diarrhea. Diarrhea is a symptom usually caused by infection, food poisoning or drug toxicity and needs to be controlled and stopped or dehydration will occur and deplete the body of its vital resources.

Virechana, on the other hand, is a natural, herb-induced purging process which automatically ceases once the accumulated *ama* and toxins are gone. The effect of the purgative herbs subsides after a short time and the patient is left feeling stronger and more vital because toxins and waste material have been eliminated. *Virechana* is a controlled process that gathers *ama* from many *pitta* locations in the body, concentrates it in the small intestine and then discharges it. It purifies *pitta* function and consequently balances and strengthens all metabolic processes.

Virechana therapy is good for all types of *pitta*-related disorders. This includes hyperacidity, colitis, urticaria, acid peptic disease, hemorrhoids, chronic headaches, some types of diabetes, allergies and skin diseases, such as acne, dermatitis, psoriasis, eczema, leprosy, leukoderma and lichen planus syndrome. It is also indicated for migraine headaches and malabsorption. *Virechana* should not be used on infants, the very elderly or pregnant women. It is also contraindicated for people who suffer from extremely weak digestion, ulcerative colitis, dehydration, emaciation and acute fever; or who pass blood with their stools.

The herbal substances which induce purgation contain a predominance of *jala* and *prithvi bhutas*. They generate a downward movement in the body, because water and earth, unlike air and fire, are heavy and gravity pulls them down. They act with varying intensity on different individuals. In sensitive people, a small amount of purgative can cause many evacuations, while others need more stimulation and may require larger doses and stronger herbs. The patient's *doshic* constitution and gastrointestinal sensitivity determine the type and amount of purgative required.

People with dominant *pitta*, who have a tendency towards frequent bowel movements with loose stools, receive mild laxatives like *nishottar* (Ipomoea Turpethum) *Kaphic* individuals, with slow bowels and heavy, sticky stools need a stronger laxative, like *amal-*

tas (Cassia Fistula) or *Indian laburnum*. Those with *vata*-dominant constitutions have a tendency towards dry, hard stools and constipation and can be harder to purge. In such cases *jaipal* (Croton Tinglium) seeds or the oil from the *eranda* (Ricinus Communis) leaf, usually known as castor oil, may be used. Some herbal purgatives combine many ingredients and work well on all constitutional types. The *Charaka Samhita* lists 315 herbal preparations that can be used for *virechana*. It is the responsibility of the trained Ayurvedic physician to select a purgative that is appropriate for each patient.

Before describing the procedure of *virechana*, I want to share an experience that demonstrates the utility of this treatment. One of my patients had a chronic *pitta* imbalance that was complicated by gallstones, chronic colitis, gastritis, hemorrhoids and an enlarged liver. I administered basic *Purvakarma* and *virechana* and followed it up with herbal *rasayana* therapy to strengthen the weakened organs and enhance the immune system. This effectively ended his digestive disorders and food allergies, removed his gallstones, and normalized his liver function.

Preparing for *Virechana*

Snehana and *swedana* treatments ready the patient for *virechana*. Full oleation is essential to dislodge the *ama* and toxins and draw them into the small intestine from the surrounding organs and tissues in the *pitta* zone. This helps assure that the purgation will be complete and comfortable. As we explained in Chapter Nine, oleation is accomplished not only by external means, but also by ingestion of oleaginous substances. Bitter *ghee* (*tikta ghrita*) is the best substance for internal oleation. Made from a decoction of over fifty-three herbs, it works on the organs in the *pitta* area, as well as all *doshic* functions throughout the body.

The meal immediately preceding *virechana* includes foods which promote secretions from the organs governed by *pitta*. Such foods are high in *pitta*-enhancing qualities — hot, spicy and sour. The purgative is taken when the meal is in the small intestine, in the second stage of *prapaka* transient digestion. This sour stage of transient digestion promotes *pitta* secretions in the mid-zone which support *virechana*. On the average, it takes about two-and-a-half hours for food to reach this phase of digestion. If the patient does not wait this long between his meal and the purgative, his food will still be in the stomach and the herbal stimulus will not be able to exert its cleansing influence on the *pitta* zone.

Once the patient has eaten, he should take it easy and refrain from physical or mental activity, which would draw blood and *doshic* activity away from the gastrointestinal tract and out to the organs and periphery of the body. If this happens, the *ama* and toxins which the preparatory procedures concentrated in the small intestine, are drawn back into the *dhatus* with the movement of the *doshas*. This severely limits *virechana*'s ability to cleanse the system.

Administration of *Virechana*

Virechana's stimulus should be used when *pitta*'s physiological activity peaks, in the hours around noon and midnight, and when *agni bhuta* is at its height of influence in the environment. For example, if *virechana* is planned for the daytime, the patient eats a *pitta*-abundant meal around 10:30 A.M. and takes the purgative two-and-a-half hours later, at 1:00 PM. It is preferable to administer the purgative at night, just before bed, when the physiology is more settled. This gives *pitta* the chance to do its work. The patient would then eat around 7:00 P.M. and take the purgative at 9:30 P.M., about the time when the *pitta* period begins.

Coordinating the timing of the meals and the purgative maximizes *pitta* secretions in the mid-zone of the body.

Several hours after taking the purgative, the patient usually begins to feel the need to move his bowels. Over the next hour the patient may have from four to ten bowel movements. The response varies from individual to individual, depending upon *doshic* constitution and the amount of *ama* in the *pitta* area. One person may have six movements while another may have fifteen. Ideally, the patient experiences at least six or eight movements. When all the toxins have been expelled from the small intestine, the urge to evacuate naturally subsides.

The fecal matter is solid at first, but progressively softens until it is entirely liquid. The patient may feel mild cramping or a burning sensation. These symptoms arise from *pitta*-related *ama* in the stool and are no cause for alarm. If severe, the patient can consume a small amount of *tikta ghrita* or medicated *ghee* to relieve them. Otherwise, he should not eat during the purging process.

The patient avoids liquids, except for some pure water with a little dried sugarcane juice (*jaggery*) and black salt (*saindhava*). The patient should drink a small amount of this or an organic electrolyte mixture after each bowel movement to replenish electrolytes and prevent dehydration. If someone dislikes the sugar and salts contained in these electrolyte solutions he can use a colloidal mineral concentrate.

For a successful *virechana*, the patient should have at least four to six bowel movements. Otherwise, the procedure should be repeated within a few hours. A small number of evacuations usually indicates that *ama* was not sufficiently purged from the small intestine. When *vata's* downward motion does not work properly, cleansing can be incomplete. As a result, the person can feel bloated in the umbilical region or hardness in the abdomen. The retention of gas and feces along with toxins and waste products might cause discomfort, and individuals might also experience itching on the skin, a metallic taste in the mouth, or nausea.

If this occurs, the patient is given hot tea made from fresh ginger or special herbal mixtures to strengthen the *ama*-reducing potency of the digestive fire. The patient should also drink warm water and apply warm compresses to his abdomen. After a few hours, *snehana* and *swedana* (oleation and heating) should be repeated and another purgative taken to complete the cleansing process.

The frequency of evacuation should be noted, as well as the quantity, color, odor, consistency and the presence of mucus, blood or parasites. By the time the cleansing is finished, the patient will have completely liquid bowel movements, which may contain some mucus. This indicates that the small intestine has been emptied and mucus from the stomach and the *kapha* zone is starting to come out. The purging process is now finished and stops automatically.

After *virechana*, the patient is cautioned to keep away from cold drinks or cold baths, because they shrink the *shrotas* or channels, aggravate *vata* and obstruct the natural flow of energy. Cold liquids also greatly tax the already weakened digestive fires. The patient is advised to rest, stay warm and relaxed, and avoid exercise or sexual activity. At this time, the patient can drink warm chamomile or licorice tea to soothe the intestinal tract. *Virechana* dramatically effects the digestive *agnis*, so it is vital for the patient to follow a special diet for several days after treatment. This allows the *agnis* to regain their normal strength and assures optimum digestion.

In very rare cases, the patient can become dehydrated or dizzy. He should continuously sip electrolytes in warm water and rest in bed until his strength returns.

After successful *virechana*, the patient feels clean, light and strong. *Pitta* is normalized, along with digestion, assimilation and appetite. Abdominal bloating and heaviness dissipate. The mind clears and the intellect sharpens. When cleansing has been complete, symptoms of *pitta* disorders, such as skin inflammation, disappear. Because it cleanses the digestive tract and improves assimilation, *virechana* enhances the benefits of *rasayana*, which rejuvenates the *dhatus*.

BASTI: THERAPEUTIC PURIFICATION AND REJUVENATION OF THE COLON

Basti therapy is perhaps the most powerful of the five main procedures of *Panchakarma*. *Charaka*, as well as many later Ayurvedic scholars, unanimously praise the value of *basti*. They say that while *vamana*, *nasya* and *virechana* together contribute fifty-percent of the benefits of *Panchakarma*, *basti* by itself, provides the other fifty-percent. The literal meaning of *Basti* is "bladder," because centuries ago, bladders made of animal skins or organs were used to administer this procedure. *Bas* carries the meaning, "to stay in place," and therefore can be understood as "that which is retained or kept inside."

Basti is the introduction of medicated liquids into the colon through the rectum. While it directly effects the colon, it is not a localized or symptomatic treatment. The colon is seldom, if ever, addressed for its own sake. Rather, it is utilized because of its vital link with all of the other organs and tissues. Consequently, *basti* has a wide-ranging influence in the body, effecting all the *doshas* and *dhatus*.

Charaka uses the analogy of a large tree with flowers, fruits, leaves, branches, bark and trunk. The whole tree depends for its nourishment on its roots. Through the roots, the tree takes in water and nutrients, which it circulates throughout its structure and transforms into its trunk, branches, leaves, etc. Thus, the root constitutes the primary organ for sustaining the life of the tree. Much like the root, the colon performs the central job of providing the nourishment that sustains all the other organs and tissues of the body.

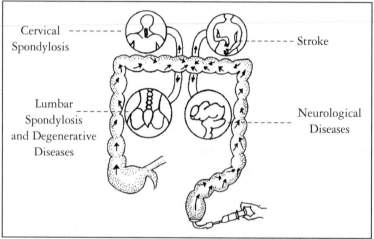

Cervical Spondylosis

Stroke

Lumbar Spondylosis and Degenerative Diseases

Neurological Diseases

Nourishment to entire body from colon
and management of various diseases

Three factors explain the colon's significant role in supporting the body:

(i) It is the main organ for absorption of nutrients from *prapaka* digestion.

(ii) The colon is the chief seat for *vata*, the prime mover of the other two *doshas*, and therefore, all physiological activities.

(iii) It constitutes the primary receptacle for waste elimination.

Basti treatments balance and nurture *vata dosha*. When *vata* functions normally, it helps bring toxins and waste matter out of the *dhatus* and eliminates them. *Vata* plays a central role in the disease process because it carries *ama* from the site of origin (in the G-I tract) to the deeper tissues where it generates disease. By managing *vata*, we gain control of the disease process before it goes into its migratory phase.

The word *basti* is frequently translated into English as "enema." However, to associate or confuse *basti* treatment with enemas misconstrues the true nature of this therapy. *Basti* differs completely from enemas or colonics in its intent, administration and effect.

Enemas treat localized symptoms of constipation by promoting evacuation. They clear feces that have collected in the rectum and sigmoid colon — the last eight to ten inches of the colon. Colonics clean accumulated fecal matter from the entire colon through repeated flushing with water. In recent years, Western practitioners of colonic therapy have begun to experiment with the addition of other substances to the water.

From the point of view of Ayurveda, emphasis on the colon as a primary eliminative pathway in the body is correct. However, repeated flushing with water, as well as the introduction of oxygen, may weaken the mucous membranes, dry the colon and further disrupt the normal eliminative work of *vata dosha*. Neither enemas nor colonics address the nutritive capability of the colon.

However, when *basti* is used in conjunction with *Panchakarma's* pre-procedures, it cleans far more than just the colon. It helps purify toxins from all over the body. Healthy colon function is not simply a matter of ridding the body of fecal material. *Vata*, with its excitable nature and drying tendency, must be nourished and pacified. In fact, the entire body can be nourished through the colon. *Basti's* palliative and nutritive qualities address these factors.

Basti introduces medicated, oily substances into the colon to be retained and absorbed by the body. It treats the entire length of the colon, from the ileocecal valve to the anus, and eliminates not only accumulated fecal matter from the colon but also *ama* and toxins from all the *dhatus*. In addition to getting rid of toxins, it restores healthy function to the colon, and through the colon nurtures and rebuilds the tissues and organs.

Therapeutic Benefits of *Basti* Therapy

Basti therapy is the most effective treatment for disorders arising from abnormal *vata*. This includes chronic constipation, low back pain, sciatica, rheumatism, gout, arthritis; and various neuromuscular disorders, such as paraplegia, hemiplegia, poliomyelitis, Alzheimer's disease, Parkinson's disease, multiple sclerosis, and dystrophy and atrophy of the nerves and muscles. It benefits epilepsy, mental retardation, and sensory dysfunction.

Vata governs and has its secondary seat in the bones. *Basti* therapy therefore also helps with disorders of *asthi dhatu*, or bone tissue, such as osteoporosis. When *vamana* and *virechana* cannot be used due to emaciation and weakness, patients can receive a combination of nutritive and cleansing *bastis*. *Basti* is generally contraindicated for infants, as well as those suffering from diarrhea, rectal bleeding, ulcerative colitis, diverticulitis, colon cancer, polyps, fever and some types of diabetes.

The effectiveness of *basti* treatment became very clear to me in the first few months of my medical practice. A man came to me with severe hiccups. They continued without stopping. Twenty-four hours a day, whether he was standing, lying down or sitting. He and his family had tried everything they could think of without success. He had become desperate since he could not eat solid food or sleep with this condition. He also reported a history of chronic hyper-acidity and colitis.

He tried homeopathy first, but when the hiccups did not stop, he consulted a number of Western physicians, including a gastroenterologist. Their examinations turned up only some gastritis and duodenitis; the medications they prescribed for these conditions did not help the hiccups. Finally he resorted to naturapathic treatments, which used medicated poultices, emetics and coffee enemas. After forty-eight hours, he had not improved. In desperation, his family decided to admit him to a Bombay hospital one day's travel from home, but no rooms were available for three days.

In the mean time, his brother-in-law heard of me and decided to give me a call. I visited the patient and gave him a thorough examination. Frankly, I felt a bit intimidated by the situation. So many doctors had tried and failed to help this man, and I was just beginning my practice and had little experience. However, I appreciated the challenge and thought to myself, "Well, let us see what this ancient knowledge can do." When I examined him, I discovered that he had not had a bowel movement in six days. His mother and wife said this was because he could not eat solid food and was taking only liquids. Though my examination confirmed the metabolic dysfunction noted by the other doctors, I felt that some key factor was being overlooked.

I deeply considered the problem, and my intuition told me to look for the answer in the *Charaka Samhita*'s description of *vata* and it's sub-functions. There it states that *vata dosha* is divided into five sub-*doshas*, (called *vayus*), each of which governs a specific type or direction of movement in the body. *Apana vayu* has a downward movement and is responsible for eliminating urine and feces. I reasoned that *apana* was not working properly because elimination was not taking place. I felt that instead of moving downward, it was, in fact, moving upward. This upward distortion of its natural movement interfered with the normal function of *udana vayu*, another sub-*dosha*, and precipitated a crisis between them. This conflict, I thought, could be the cause of the hiccups.

I remembered from the texts that *basti* treatment is always prescribed for any acute *vata* imbalance. I explained to the man and his family what I thought should be done, but they could not understand how an "enema" would help. Luckily, the mother-in-law was somewhat familiar with Ayurvedic treatment and said, "OK, let's try it. If it works we will not have to travel 600 miles to Bombay."

First I administered a water-based, cleansing *nirooha basti*. After three hours, I administered an oil-based, nourishing *anuwasan basti*. Three hours later, I administered another *nirooha basti*. I went to see him the next morning and found that there was no change in his condition. His family was disappointed that nothing had yet happened. However, I was confident that the theory was sound, so they allowed me to continue treatment.

I administered an *anuwasan basti*, and after three hours, another *nirooha basti*. Then I went home. When I came back in the evening to administer one more *anuwasan basti*, the patient greeted me at the door. He said, "You are a great doctor! After you left I had a bowel movement. Stone-like fecal matter came out, and then suddenly, after that evacuation, my hiccups stopped. Thank you!" Needless to say, I was happy and even a little surprised at the success of this uncomplicated treatment.

When I went home, I pondered the fact that this man had experienced such wonderful results in such a short period of time. The treatment was so simple. The previous treatments had concentrated on the inflammation of the upper G-I tract. They did not consider the possibility that wastes and toxins remained in the patient's body and impaired the normal functions of *vata*.

I did not specifically treat the gastritis or the hiccups. I treated *apana vayu*, restoring its natural downward direction and thus the normal peristalsis of the colon. This reduced the bloating and gas and eliminated the *malas* that had accumulated in his colon. With *apana vayu* flowing in its proper direction and some of the toxins removed from the colon, the other sub-functions of *vata* regained their correct functioning. As soon as the hyperactivity of *udana vayu* settled down, the hiccups ceased.

Another example of the effectiveness of *basti* therapy came from treating a man who had suffered a stroke six months before coming to see me. His left side was completely paralyzed. He had been diagnosed with a type of flaccid paralysis hemiplegia and his family had been told that nothing could be done except maintain his vital functions. The doctors suggested physiotherapy, but doubted whether it would have much effect. The bedridden patient received six months of physiotherapy, but his condition showed no improvement.

He came to my clinic in a wheelchair and could not even lift his hand. The Ayurvedic texts generally attribute such conditions to a block in *vata*'s movement. Accordingly, I put him on a special regimen, including *snehana*, *pinda swedana*, *nasya* and a type of *basti* therapy designed to strengthen *mamsa dhatu* and restore neuromuscular function. In the two years that he has been under treatment, he has recovered almost total mobility and coordination. Today he walks well on his own, although he occasionally needs to pay attention when walking fast or lifting. He returned to work and now leads a normal life.

Because of poor nutrition and physical stress, many patients in India suffer from spondylosis, an inflammation of the cervical or lumbar vertebrae and a herniation of the discs. Even with surgery, many people become physically incapacitated or experience chronic pain. I have repeatedly found that *Panchakarma* with an emphasis on *basti* quickly reduces or eliminates the pain and muscle spasms, and in most cases, restores spinal mobility. However, I have not yet determined to what extent degenerated discs can be restored, and it will take years of research to do so.

I have also had great success treating sciatica-types of disorders with *basti* therapy. Not only do these patients return to work free from pain, but, in many cases, no longer require surgery. Such spinal diseases usually result from debilitated *asthi* and *majja dhatus*. The spinal inflammation common to these bone and marrow disorders is due to an *ama* accumulation that severely blocks *vata*'s work in that area.

Since *vata* governs bone and bone marrow, *bastis* — particularly oil-predominant *bastis* — are an essential part of the treatment program. Oil's slow, heavy qualities directly counteract the dry, rapid and mobile qualities of deranged *vata*. These patients need thorough internal and external oleation. This removes *ama* from the spine, corrects *vata* dysfunction and reestablishes pain-free mobility. I have also used this therapy with extremely good results in cases of poliomyelitis and muscular dystrophy.

TYPES OF *BASTI* THERAPY

Basti fulfills many needs, so the type of *basti* used during *Panchakarma* varies according to the intended purpose of the treatment. One type of *basti* eliminates the *ama* that has gathered in the colon from throughout the body. Another normalizes *vata* function. If the prime mover is out of balance, everything is out of balance. Once *vata* has returned to normal functioning, *basti* therapy is then used to nourish and revitalize the *dhatus*.

It is by far the most important procedure in *Panchakarma* because of its versatility. *Vamana* and *virechana* fulfill one primary objective — cleansing the body of toxins. *Basti*, however, accomplishes this, as well as two additional purposes. Palliative *bastis* balance the *doshas*, reduce symptoms and make the patient more comfortable. Nutritive *bastis* nourish and rebuild the *dhatus*, strengthen their activity, and restore and strengthen immunity. No other single treatment provides such direct and far-reaching benefits.

Although every major classical Ayurvedic text regards *basti* therapy as a major curative treatment, several different systems for classifying them have evolved. The most comprehensive system of classification concerns the site of administration. The next categorizes *basti* by its function. The last method refers to the frequency and duration of *bastis*. We'll discuss all of these systems, beginning with the broadest.

1. *Basti* Classified By Site of Administration

The first major classification scheme refers to the administration site and the primary organs receiving treatment. It recognizes four areas:

Pakwashaya gata basti. Medicated liquids sent through the anus and rectum into the colon

Uttara basti. Medicated liquids sent through the vagina and cervix to cleanse and nourish the uterus

Mutrashaya gata basti. Medicated liquids introduced into the penis and urethra to treat the male genital and urinary organs

Vranagata basti. Cleansing and medicated liquids used to irrigate and heal abscesses or wounds

The Ayurvedic texts describe one final class of nutritive, palliative *basti*, which is not administered internally through the rectum, vagina, penis, etc., but rather externally in localized areas of the body, such as the lower back or eyes. Even though they are not introduced into the body, they are still called *basti* because the medicated, lubricated substances are retained in areas of the body for a period of time.

Four types of external *bastis* are classified according to their site of administration:

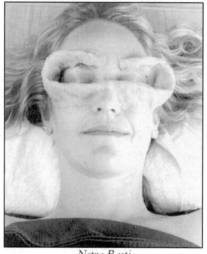

Netra Basti

Netra basti or *netra tarpana*, applies medicated *ghee* to the eyes. The *ghee* is contained by a dam constructed around the eye sockets, made of the dough from black gram flour. *Netra basti* is highly nourishing for the eyes, removes eye strain and improves vision.

Katti basti means "retained on the lower back." It applies medicated oils in a container of black gram dough built around the lumbosacral area. This form of external *basti* particularly benefits muscle spasm and rigidity of the lower spine and strengthens the bone tissue in that area.

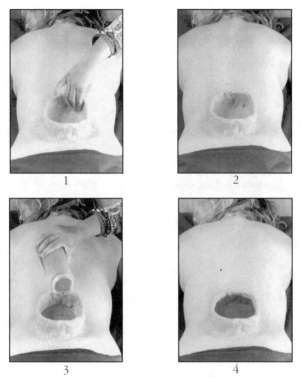

Katti Basti

Uro basti means "retained on the chest and heart area." It uses medicated oils in a container — also constructed of black gram dough — around the heart. It reduces pain in the sternum area and strengthens the heart.

Shiro basti is administered on the head through the use of a specialized leather container resembling a hat. This type of *basti* improves the functioning of *prana vayu* and revitalizes sensory functioning. It also promotes *kaphagenic* secretions in the para-nasal sinus zone which reduce vascular congestion in the brain. *Shiro basti* is extremely useful in vascular headaches, schizophrenia, obsessive-compulsive disorders, memory loss, disorientation, glaucoma and sinus headaches.

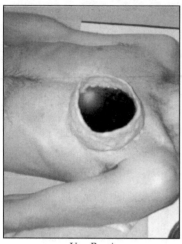

Uro Basti

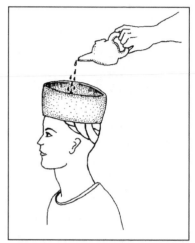

Shiro Basti

2. *Basti* Classified by Function

While *Charaka* developed and presented *basti* therapy in great detail, his knowledge provides general guidelines which allow experienced and well-trained Ayurvedic physicians to adapt treatment to their patients' needs. Following *Charaka*, two other classical teachers, *Sushruta* and *Vagabhata*, divided *basti* therapy into nine types, based on their specific functions in the body. Each type has its own indications, contraindications and variations. Briefly described, they are:

1. *Shodhana basti* cleanses and detoxifies. It is divided into strong treatments which penetrate to the deeper *dhatus*, and mild treatments, which work on the more superficial level of the *dhatus*. *Nirooha* offers the prime example of this form of therapy.

2. *Utkleshana basti*, meaning "promoting secretions in the colon," promotes the liquefaction of *ama* and *mala* in the colon. It helps the colon expel them. Similar to Western enemas, this *basti* increases colonic peristalsis, producing rapid elimination of the feces.

3. *Shamana basti* is palliative. It restores *doshic* performance, reduces symptoms and allows the patient to feel better. In cases of rectal bleeding or dysentery, the immediate objective is to stop the symptoms. For example, *pichha basti*, which uses astringent herbs, shrinks the capillaries or *shrotas* and stops the bleeding or peristalsis, ending the symptoms.

4. *Lekhana basti*, meaning "strong and penetrating," resembles *shodhana basti*, but is stronger in its effects and generally much larger in volume. It is particularly useful for *kapha* and *meda dhatu* disorders, where excess fatty substances have accumulated that need to be eliminated, as in obesity and arteriosclerosis.

5. *Bruhan basti* nourishes. Highly nutritious substances are used to balance and strengthen the *dhatus* and their metabolism, and increase the body's resistance to infectious diseases. *Anuwasan* provides the prime example of *bruhan basti*. There are also nutritive *bastis*, like *ksheer bastis*, which are medicated decoctions made with fresh, whole milk. These *bastis* are very effective in regenerating the *dhatus* and are specifically used to tone the muscles (*mamsa*) and reduce atrophy and emaciation. In addition, there are *bruhan bastis* which use honey, *ghee*, or the juices from meat, bone marrow and herbs, which have a highly nutritive value.

6. *Snehana basti* is similar to *anuwasan* because it is prepared only from oleated substances, but is larger. Because of its size, it has a greater lubricating effect on both the colon and the body in general. It has a strongly pacifying influence on *vata* and is particularly useful in cracking of joints and for those who have very dry skin or who are emaciated.

7. *Rasayana basti* rejuvenates and can be prepared to rebuild and strengthen either specific *dhatus* or the whole body. *Bastis* containing both *ashwagandha* and *shatavari* improve *asthi dhatu* metabolism and have a particularly beneficial effect in osteoporosis.

8. *Vajikarana basti* treats infertility; it increases virility and fertility and gives vigor and vitality to the body. *Jivaneyam basti*, for instance, helps fertility by improving the function of *shukra dhatu*, the reproductive tissue.

9. *Matra basti* can be given any time of the day, and is particularly useful to pacify *vata* aggravation resulting from travel, exercise or stress. It is an oil *basti* that can be self-administered in very small amounts, usually about 30 ml. or 1-1/2 ounces.

3. *Basti* Classified By Frequency and Duration

Charaka describes three additional *basti* classifications which are based on specific treatment regimens: *karma basti*, *kala basti* and *yoga basti*. They address serious conditions arising from *vata* derangement, and involve various alternations of nourishing and cleansing *bastis* for a set number of days, finishing with several nourishing *bastis*.

Karma basti comprises a month-long treatment and is given to people who have *vata*-dominant constitutions and *vata*-related disorders. It begins with *anuwasan basti* and alternates with *nirooha basti* for twenty-five consecutive days. The thirty-day program ends with five days of *anuwasan bastis*.

Kala basti lasts for fifteen days and is used mainly for patients with *pitta*-dominant constitutions and *vata* disorders. It starts with an *anuwasan basti*, which then alternates with *nirooha bastis* for ten or twelve days and concludes with three or five days of *anusawan bastis*.

Yoga basti, given for eight days, suits *kaphic* patients with *vata* diseases. It first gives *anuwasan basti*, and alternates three times with *nirooha*. It concludes with two days of *anuwasan*.

TYPE OF *BASTIS* USED IN PANCHAKARMA

Due to the importance of the colon's eliminative and rejuvenating functions, *Panchakarma* largely employs *pakwashaya gata basti*. We will now discuss the two main types of *pakwashaya gata basti* given during this therapy. They are called *nirooha* and *anuwasan basti*. All other *bastis*, whether based on administrative site or specific purpose, serve only an adjunctive function in *Panchakarma*.

Nirooha Basti: Cleansing *Basti*

Nirooha, which means "that which gets eliminated," cleanses toxins from the *dhatus* and removes naturally accumulated *malas* from the colon. The *Charaka Samhita* has indicated that this *shodhana* type of *basti* is capable of cleansing the entire body. These *bastis* primarily, but not exclusively, use water-based decoctions of purifying herbs. The quantity of liquid administered is approximately 400 ml. (1-3/4 cups), though the dosage may vary from individual to individual.

The quantity is always less than in enemas, since the *basti*'s efficacy and specific action is not based on the volume of the liquids, but on the effects of the herbs. In *nirooha*, or purifying *bastis*, the liquid is retained in the colon for approximately forty-eight minutes. During this time, some of the ingredients get absorbed and their purifying influence moves throughout the body. The rest gets expelled along with fecal matter and toxins.

Nirooha bastis are given in a series of treatments over a period of several days. These *bastis*, along with the preparatory procedures, allow the cleansing process to reach deeper and deeper into the tissues with each passing day. The benefits resemble those which *snehana* (oleation) produces in the *dhatus*.

The first day of this *basti* treatment cleanses the colon of *ama* and *mala*. The second day of *nirooha* balances and nourishes *vata*, producing increased mental calm and clarity. Because the *vata* zone has now been cleared, the third day pulls out *ama* and toxins from the *pitta* zone. This balances and nourishes *pitta* function and, in turn, purifies and strengthens both *rasa* and *rakta dhatu*. The patient experiences more strength as *rasa* improves, and better skin color and texture as *rakta* gains in health.

On the fourth and fifth days of administration, toxins get pulled out of the *kapha* area. *Kapha* resides in two major sites, other than the stomach: *mamsa* (muscles) and *meda* (adipose tissue), and this cleansing automatically purifies and strengthens both of them. On the sixth and seventh days, the *basti's* benefits reach the deeper *dhatus*, *asthi* (bone) and *majja* (bone marrow), and the eighth day works on *shukra* (semen or ovum). This sequential cleansing process stimulates the natural absorptive and eliminative functions of the colon to remove *ama* and *malas* from all the tissues of the body.

The colon demonstrates an amazing absorptive capacity, and the rejuvenating and cleansing herbs administered through *basti* easily penetrate the body and bring their healing influence from the more superficial levels of the *dhatus'* to its deeper structures. It is this type of cleansing action that led *Charaka* to exclaim, "*Basti* works from head to toe."

Anuwasan Basti: Nourishing *Basti*

Anuwasan basti, the second major type of *pakwashaya gata basti*, has as its purpose to nourish the body. It does so through the application of herbalized oils. Oil naturally lubricates and nourishes the *dhatus*, an effect which is opposite to the drying and wasting influence of excessive *vata*. Therefore, this class of *bastis* is particularly successful in the treatment of *vata* disorders. Because the disease process almost always involves some *vata* derangement, the lubricating and strengthening actions of *anuwasan bastis* are helpful in all situations calling for *basti* therapy.

Anuwasan bastis are usually administered after a cleansing course of *nirooha bastis* to insure that *vata dosha* is operating properly. They not only restore health to the colon, but also lubricate and nourish all the *dhatus*. This counteracts the debilitating influence of *ama* and toxins on the tissues and helps restore them to normality, the primary purpose of *anuwasan basti*.

The word *anuwasan* refers to "that which is to remain in the body for a while." For this type of *basti*, it is optimum if it can be retained in the body for a longer period of time in order to have its intended effect. Three to six hours is the ideal retention time. If it is administered in the evening, it is best if it can be held overnight. Occasionally, because of a reflexive colonic response, the patient will not be able to keep even a small *anuwasan basti*. Patients are instructed never to strain to hold any *basti*, but to go with their natural response. In such cases, a second oil *basti* should be given immediately.

Bastis are always applied slowly, but *anuwasan* should be introduced extremely slowly, ideally, a drop at a time. This is particularly important for individuals with irritable bowel syndrome. Slow administration reduces the possibility that a hyperactive colon will go into a reflexive response and reject the *basti*, and insures that the *basti*'s nourishing ingredients will soothe and restore normal function to the colon.

Anuwasan bastis are prepared in a wide variety of ways, depending on the specific nutritive requirement. They can benefit neuromuscular disorders, in which every *dhatu* is impaired, including muscles, bone, bone marrow and nerve tissue.

Preparing for *Basti* Therapy

As with all *Panchakarma* purification procedures, proper preparation is crucial for successful *basti* treatment. First, *snehana* and *swedana* must loosen *ama* and open the body's channels so that it can be moved out. This greatly aids the effectiveness of both the cleansing and nourishing *bastis*. *Bastis* are always administered immediately after oleation and sudation (heating). Because of these preparatory procedures, the patient feels calm and settled and his *shrotas* (channels) are dilated. This facilitates the work of the *doshas*, which is to remove *ama* from the colon and deliver nutritive substances to the *dhatus*.

Basti ingredients are freshly prepared. A typical *anuwasan basti* consists of approximately 60 ml. (3 ounces) of herbalized sesame oil. *Nirooha bastis* contain primarily herbal decoctions of water with a small amount of oil. A typical *nirooha basti* contains 400 ml. (1-3/4 cups) of a water decoction of *dashmoola*, a standard preparation consisting of a mixture of ten different herbal roots (plus additional herbs depending on the condition), 30 ml. (1-1/2 ounces) of sesame oil, a little honey and a pinch of black salt (*saindhava*). The black salt is added to increase secretions in the colon. The attending physician adjusts the exact ingredients, the ratio of oil to water and the total amount of liquid, depending on the patient's *doshic* make-up, the condition of the colon, the strength of the digestive *agnis* and the specific disorder being treated.

Basti Administration

To facilitate the movement of the *basti* fluids from the rectum up through the descending colon, patient always lies on the left side when receiving *bastis*. The patient extends his left leg, while bending his right knee and drawing it up towards the chest. This makes the anal opening more accessible to the nurse or physician administering the *bastis*. The patient's head should be supported on a pillow and he should be warm and relaxed.

The *basti* temperature must be near or at body temperature to increase the body's receptivity to treatment. The decoction is drawn up into a rectal syringe and introduced into the rectum through a thin rubber catheter. Both the anal opening and the catheter are lubricated to allow easier access. With the permission of the patient, the doctor or nurse introduces the catheter, slowly and gently, about six inches into the rectum while the patient inhales deeply. After the *basti*, the patient lies on his back and rests for ten to twenty minutes. This quiet time gives the body the chance to make the most effective use of the *basti*.

Because of its small volume, *anuwasan basti* can be easily

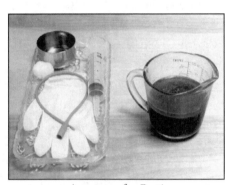

Apparatus for *Basti*

retained for a long period of time. However, with *nirooha basti*, the patient is more likely to feel the urge to defecate within forty-five minutes to an hour and, in some cases, sooner. In *nirooha*, the *ama* which the *doshas* drew into the colon is eliminated along with much of the *basti* fluid and fecal matter.

In rare cases, the body holds *nirooha basti* for as long as six to eight hours before the patient has the urge to defecate. This is not desirable, since this *basti* is supposed to cleanse. However, when *vata* is highly deranged, the colon can become extremely dry. Much of the water in the *nirooha basti* is absorbed to compensate for that dryness, in spite of the cleansing and eliminative herbs used. In such cases the patient must receive a *snehana basti* (large oil *basti*) before any further cleansing *bastis* are attempted. The *snehana basti* nourishes *vata dosha*, lubricates the colon and starts peristalsis.

The time of *basti* administration is noted along with the time of each subsequent bowel movement. It is often not possible for the physician to do this, so the patient is instructed to observe and note the frequency, color, consistency, odor and other signs which can show the physician whether *ama* is present and what type of *ama* is being eliminated.

Treatment Regimen

The Ayurvedic physician always closely monitors the patient's response to *basti* treatments. He then makes adjustments in the type of *basti*, its oil and water content, the specific herbal decoctions used and the number of *bastis* given. Most patients gain greatest benefit from a series of *bastis* which alternate *nirooha* with *anuwasan*.

Based on information presented in the *Charaka Samhita*, several regimens which alternate herbal water decoctions with oil *bastis* are employed. The specific regimen depends on the constitution of the patient and the condition of the colon. A *nirooha* decoction is often applied for two consecutive days and then followed by an oil-based *anuwasan basti* on the third. If there is greater need for cleansing, *nirooha bastis* can be given for three days, followed by oil on the fourth.

In most cases, this type of treatment schedule, followed for eight to ten days, cleanses *ama* and *mala* from the *dhatus* and assists the rebuilding of *dhatu* structures. This regimen restores normal balance to the *doshas* and the *dhatus*.

It is essential to always end treatment with *anuwasan basti*. This guarantees that *vata* is operating properly and that the colon is left lubricated and nourished. When properly administered, *basti* treatment does not interfere with normal intestinal flora and strengthens the function of the mucous membranes lining the colon.

Bastis have proven remarkably successful in treating situations that have not responded to any other form of therapy. Their power and efficacy as a treatment modality have gone largely unrecognized by modern medicine. When the vital functions of *vata dosha* are not understood, it is easy to overlook the tremendous absorptive power of the colon. As a consequence, modern medicine has failed to take advantage of the colon as an important route for the administration of medicines and nutrients.

Modern application of *basti* therapy confirms the knowledge in the ancient classical Ayurvedic texts: Of all the possible routes of administration, the colon most readily absorbs substances into the body. In addition, because the colon is so intimately linked to the body's tissues, it is the best organ to eliminate toxins and *mala*.

An example from my own clinical practice dramatically demonstrates the utility of *basti* therapy. Some years ago a young girl was brought to me by her parents. She had cancer and had been treated by chemotherapy to no avail. She had grown progressively weaker until her body could not assimilate any medications or food taken orally. By the time she came to my clinic, her condition had severely deteriorated.

I decided as a last resort to use the colon to supply nutrition to her emaciated body. She was put on a course of *basti* treatment that alternated nourishing *bruhan bastis* with oleating *snehana bastis*. Her body responded well to this treatment. In a short time she regained her strength and was able to accept food by mouth.

This experience proved to me how powerful the colon is as an organ of assimilation. It can be counted on to absorb and utilize nutritive and medicated substances when all else fails. This approach not only provided her body with desperately needed nutrition, but also normalized her metabolism by correcting *vata* function and removing *ama*. It quickly restored her ability to take food and medicines by mouth. As I stated in the introduction of this book, it has been gratifying to find the solutions to difficult medical problems consistently and clearly elaborated in the ancient Ayurvedic texts, some of which are over 5,000 years old.

RAKTAMOKSHANA: THERAPEUTIC WITHDRAWAL OF BLOOD

Thousands of years ago, *Charaka* wrote the oldest and most extensive text of Ayurveda, thoroughly explaining the science of Ayurveda. In this treatise, he also delineated the five *karmas* or major procedures of *vamana, nasya, virechana*, cleansing and nourishing *bastis* for purifying and rejuvenating the body. He is consequently considered to be the father of Ayurvedic internal medicine.

After *Charaka, Sushruta* is perhaps the most important commentator on the "science of life." *Sushruta* is known as the father of Ayurvedic surgery because his focus was more narrowly defined by treatment methodologies used in critical disease situations. Many of the surgical procedures and instruments which he describes in his scholarly writings thousands of years ago have been rediscovered in the last 150 years by Western medical science.

Although Ayurveda favors prevention wherever possible, traumatic invasive surgery is advised in certain acute cases. *Sushruta's* extensive experience in the examination of blood during the course of surgery enabled him to gain a deep understanding of the relationship of the blood to *rakta dhatu, pitta dosha* and diseases associated with their toxicity and malfunction. He subsequently combined the two main types of *basti* discussed by *Charaka* into one category and added *raktamokshana* — the therapeutic withdrawal of blood from the body — as the fifth major procedure used in *Panchakarma* therapy.

Sushruta attributed particular importance to the blood because it performed the important job of providing transportation within the body. He noted that when *ama* or toxins collected, they were circulated throughout the body with the blood. Through extensive observation of the blood, he identified several different types of blood toxemia based on *doshic* imbalance. He devised *raktamokshana* as a purification treatment to be used when excess toxins are being carried in the blood to the periphery of the body.

Although *raktamokshana* is the most limited of the five major procedures, it provides a rapid and sometimes dramatic reduction of symptoms in certain acute disorders, especially where time is a critical factor. The other procedures are much more comprehensive in their scope and are applied after *raktamokshana* is completed in order to provide deep cleansing of *ama* from the tissues and thereby eliminate the actual disease process. ·

Rakta dhatu and *pitta dosha* are closely associated and their functions interrelated. The blood, which represents *rakta dhatu*, is formed and regulated by the liver, spleen and bone marrow, which perform *pitta*-related work. For this reason, when toxins appear due to excess *pitta*, they concentrate in the blood. Examination of the blood can then provide significant diagnostic information about the condition of *pitta* and its associated organs.

When excessive *pitta*-related *ama* exists in the blood, it gets transported to the body's periphery, where it often produces characteristic symptoms like skin inflammation or skin hypersensitivity. Acute symptoms can usually be relieved within a few hours by simply removing a small amount of toxic blood from the affected area. Once *ama* is gone, *rakta* metabolism improves, and the blood can perform its job efficiently. When toxins associated with *pitta* are eliminated, *pitta* function regains balance.

Raktamokshana successfully treats blood-related diseases, including many types of skin disorders: chronic itching, eczema, urticaria, rashes, and leukoderma. It is also indicated for enlarged liver or spleen, gout and some types of headaches and hypertension. *Raktamokshana* is most often prescribed towards the end of summer and during autumn, when *pitta* tends to become aggravated due to *agni bhuta's* dominance in the environment. It is contraindicated for infants, pregnant or menstruating women, the aged, and those with anemia, edema, leukemia, cirrhosis of the liver, and any bleeding in the body.

Administration of *Raktamokshana*

Snehana and *swedana* do not have to precede *raktamokshana*. On the day of treatment, the patient simply lies on a table and a small amount of blood is withdrawn intravenously. In ancient times, several different methods were used, depending on the patient's *doshic* constitution. Today, we use a sterile syringe. This procedure should always be performed under qualified medical supervision. The venipuncture is sealed by medicated gauze and a pressure bandage is applied for a short time. After approximately one hour, the patient can get up and leave.

The blood is examined for color, smell, consistency, viscosity and clotting characteristics. The specific characteristics of the blood will indicate the quality of function in the *pitta* zone.

In my clinical practice I have seen some remarkable results from the use of this procedure. A patient once came to me with oozing eczema on his whole body and an extremely swollen face. Because he had unusually high blood pressure, I could not immediately use the other cleansing procedures. Instead I performed *raktamokshana*, removing 80 cc. of blood from his body. Within six hours the oozing and itching stopped; his skin, which had previously been a darkish gray, returned to a more normal color and all the swelling disappeared from his face and body.

Because the toxins in his peripheral circulation were quickly removed, all his symptoms were reduced within a short period of time. After this, he was put on a *Purvakarma* regimen, followed by the major *karmas* of *vamana*, *virechana*, and *bastis*, and he recovered completely. With this thorough cleansing, as well as diet and lifestyle changes to avoid future toxicity, he has remained free from these unpleasant skin disorders.

In another case, a patient who suffered from migraines came to my clinic with a severe headache. Fifteen minutes after performing *raktamokshana* on a point called the *shankha marma* in the temporal-occipital region of his head, the headache was gone and he did not have to take pain medication.

I offer you these anecdotal experiences to demonstrate the effectiveness of removing toxins directly from the bloodstream by withdrawing blood. It can be used in most situations where symptoms must be reduced quickly, and where the cause of symptoms lies in a derangement in the function of *rakta dhatu*.

When *raktamokshana* is contraindicated but symptoms indicate that the blood is toxic and needs to be cleansed, Ayurveda employs *shamana* or palliative therapies. These include adjustments in diet, and the use of specific herbs to cleanse the blood. In Ayurveda, the blood is said to be the carrier of *ayu*, or life, so its condition directly influences the four parts of life: *atma* (soul), *manas* (mind), *indriyas* (senses) and *sharira* (body). Good blood, free from toxins and waste products, sustains life and helps maintain the physiological equilibrium necessary for health.

CLINCAL EXPERIENCE IN *PANCHAKARMA* THERAPY

Earlier in the chapter I gave some examples from my clinical experiences regarding the healing potential of *nasya*, *virechana*, *vamana* and *basti*. However, treatment of most diseased conditions demands that these procedures be applied in unison in order to eradicate the root cause of the disease. The following case histories address specific conditions:

Obesity

Obesity responds well to *Panchakarma* therapy. Removing *ama* and excess fat from *meda dhatu* improves fat metabolism. I remember treating a thirty-two year old gentleman with a serious case of obesity. I used a treatment prescribed by the ancient texts, called *udvartana*. In this procedure, a dry, herbalized powder is vigorously massaged into the skin in place of oil during *snehana* to enliven *meda dhatu's* metabolism. In addition, a special type of *basti* called *lekhana basti* was used to activate and then eliminate excess fat. Special medicated *nasyas* were also employed to remove *kapha*-related *ama* from the head region, which helped to restore the patient's normal endocrinal functions.

Menstrual Irregularity

My wife, Dr. Shalmali Joshi, is also an Ayurvedic physician, specializing in women's health and gynecology, and has applied *Panchakarma* to a wide variety of gynecological problems. A woman came to Shalmali for obesity. Shalmali's diagnosis indicated that the weight problem was due to secondary amenorrhea — the sudden cessation of the menstrual cycle caused by impairment of *rasa dhatu agni* — which naturally causes an accumulation of *kapha*. The woman received *vamana*, *virechana* and *basti*, which rekindled her *agni*; her menstrual cycles returned to normal and her weight problem disappeared.

Infertility

We remember a woman who consulted with Shalmali about the inability to conceive. Upon examination, my wife learned that the woman had irregular menstrual cycles, hormonal imbalances and unpredictable ovulation. She had been treated with Western medicine but the prescription only seemed to complicate her condition.

Shalmali administered a series of *bastis* and *nasyas* which restored hormonal balance and menstrual regularity. She then gave *uttara bastis*, medicated substances designed to cleanse and nourish the uterus. Shortly after completing these treatments, the woman was able to conceive and subsequently gave birth to a healthy little girl.

Arthritis

Arthritis is considered to be an auto-immune disorder, but Western medical science does not understand its causes. As a result, only palliative types of treatments are available. However, when the Ayurvedic texts were written thousands of years ago, they described a disease called *amavat*, in which *ama* clogs the *shrotas* or channels of the body and restricts *vata*'s motion. This produces loss of mobility in the joints, resulting in pain and swelling, or what we currently call rheumatoid arthritis. *Panchakarma* therapy can control this disorder, and, if treated in its early stages, reverse it. It cleanses toxins from the *shrotas* so that *vata* can again carry *prana* and nutrition to *asthi dhatu*, or bone.

I have treated many patients with this illness and have found this therapy to be successful in eighty to ninety percent of the cases. My approach to treating rheumatic patients is always first to strengthen their digestive *agni* and improve their digestion, assimilation and elimination; and, secondly, to strengthen the immune system.

The value of this two-pronged approach is dramatically illustrated in the case of a man who came all the way from Los Angeles to my clinic in Nagpur. His condition was so crippling that even his mind was affected and he was forced to take early retirement. After two months of treatment, he recuperated so remarkably that he undertook a tour of India without a recurrence of his symptoms. Upon his return to Los Angeles, he resumed his full professional responsibilities.

Parkinson's Disease

I recall the case of a fifty-eight year old man who had suffered from Parkinson's disease for seventeen years. When he first came to my clinic, he could only walk with the support of two people. He was taking the maximum prescribable dosage of dopamine to reduce his tremors and increase his muscular coordination.

This type of disease is a *vata* disorder involving degeneration of *majja dhatu* (bone marrow), and treatment centers on *vata* pacification. Initially, I gave him *snehana*, *nasya* and *bastis* to cleanse and calm the *vata* zone, and then switched to nourishing and rejuvenating treatments like *pinda swedana*, *Pishinchhali* and *ksheer bastis* to nourish *mamsa* (muscle) and *majja* (bone marrow) *dhatus*. In three months he was walking without support and I was able to reduce his dopamine intake by one-half. While not totally healed, he was so improved that he undertook a long journey to Northern India by himself.

Other Degenerative Disorders

I have treated many other degenerative disorders, such as multiple sclerosis, muscular dystrophy, epilepsy, mental retardation and various connective tissue disorders, and have found that they all respond well to *Panchakarma* therapy. In severe cases, I have not been able to completely cure the disease, but I have been able to stop its progression and alleviate some of the debilitating symptoms.

I am confident that cancer can respond well to *shodhana* therapy although I have not had much experience treating this disease because cancer patients tend to come to me at the last stages of their disease and are essentially incurable. From the Ayurvedic point of view, cancer is a condition of depleted *agni* or vital force that occurs because *vata* functioning becomes severely deranged. One of *Panchakarma*'s main effects is to restore normal *vata* function and improve the vital force. The key is to treat this disease in its early stages.

Another disease condition which I feel can respond well to *Panchakarma* therapy is that of AIDS. In Ayurveda, this disease is called *Ojakshaya*, or the "depletion of *ojas* from the body." *Ojas* is defined as the refined product of the seven stages of *dhatu* metabolism. It constitutes the most crucial factor in the strength and vitality of the immune system. When the *dhatu agnis* become weak, the metabolic processes within each *dhatu* get depleted, which prevents *ojas* from forming. This in turn impairs the ability of the immune system to attack and control viral growth in the body.

The conditions that are judged incurable by Western medicine have, in most cases, taken decades to manifest their symptoms. Thus, it is only reasonable to expect that it may take some time for *Panchakarma* to root out their causes. Some of the cases recounted above entailed a series of treatments to accomplish an improvement or cure. However, in my experience, due to the fast pace of life in the West, few people have the time to undergo extended *Panchakarma* treatments. Consequently, the hundreds of treatments in India which I have given to Western patients have only been of one week duration. Nonetheless, I have witnessed that many conditions respond very favorably to these shorter treatment regimens. I will share the following anecdotes to demonstrate what can be accomplished in such a short amount of time.

Chronic Fatigue Syndrome

In India I have seen many Western patients suffering with Chronic Fatigue Syndrome. According to the Ayurvedic model, this disorder manifests because of weak digestive *agni* and blocked *shrotas* which inhibit both *prana* (life-force) and nutritive substances from reaching the *dhatus*. When the tissues are undernourished and the vital force and immunity grow weak, viruses and bacteria gain a foothold, causing patients to feel constantly tired and vulnerable to infections. Even with a single eight-day *Panchakarma* program, a vast majority of these patients show a significant change in their energy level and digestion. When followed with an appropriate diet and lifestyle, they can regain their normal level of activity.

I treated a psychologist with long-term Chronic Fatigue Syndrome, who had lost his ability to work. After a week of *Panchakarma*, many of his symptoms disappeared; his tiredness abated and he was able to return to professional duties.

Insomnia and Depression

Insomnia and anxiety depression are common problems associated with *vata* imbalance. With *Panchakarma* and a proper diet and behavior regimen, I have seen dramatic changes with these patients. A middle-aged woman from New Mexico, suffering from insomnia, restlessness, lack of focus and depression for several years, asked for treatment. I designed an eight-day *vata*-pacifying *Panchakarma* program for her that positively transformed her sleep, mental balance and behavior. After six months, she returned for a follow-up and told me that she had experienced a miracle. For the first time in years, she slept soundly throughout the night and finally finished a documentary project which she had been working on for a long time. She then described the best effect of *Panchakarma*: She felt vitally connected to her source of consciousness within and said that she never wanted to lose this experience.

Chronic Pain

Another female patient came to me who had been suffering with pain throughout her body for, she said, "as long as I can remember." In addition, she reported chronic constipation and strong allergies to certain foods. This informed me that *ama* had been overloading all her *dhatus* for many years, and that this was the source of her chronic pain. *Ama* had also adversely affected *vata*'s functioning in her colon, destroying its motility. The week-long *Panchakarma* treatment expelled the toxins from her body, and as a result, she noticed a profound relief from pain and no longer resorted to the use of analgesics. Her digestion and elimination also improved so markedly that her food allergies disappeared.

Bronchial Asthma

I remember a fifty-year-old lady with acute bronchial asthma. For twenty-five years, she had depended on cortical steroids, bronchodilators and nebulizers, and had repeatedly been admitted to hospitals for her condition. I told her that an eight-day *Panchakarma* regimen would help her, but that her type of illness really demanded a series of such treatments. She agreed and within a six-month period, underwent three weeks of *Panchakarma*. The result is that she now no longer uses steroids or nebulizers nor does she have problems with breathing. Her weight decreased and, for the first time in years, she feels energetic and enthusiastic.

Irritable Bowel Syndrome

I saw a physician who had suffered from irritable bowel syndrome for three years. This condition was initially caused by amoebic dysentery contracted during visits to Asia and had generated complications involving acute digestive disorders, food allergies and severe skin rashes. With one eight-day treatment regimen, almost all his symptoms disappeared. After six months, he returned to see me and commented that even after a stressful period, which included his father's death, the symptoms did not return.

With each of these experiences my knowledge and confidence has grown. Over the years, I have had the opportunity to successfully apply the principles of *Panchakarma* therapy to many types of degenerative disorders. I have put into practice with my patients the instructions contained in the ancient texts, and have seen the effectiveness of this approach demonstrated again and again.

Research by Gabriel Cousens, M.D., has demonstrated *Panchakarma*'s ability to reduce organ and blood toxicity*. Dr. Hari Sharma of Ohio State University has explored the use of *Panchakarma* to remove blockages in coronary arteries, and has found remarkable results. Maharishi Ayurveda has also been very active in doing research on this healing modality. It is my hope for the future that many more medical scientists will become active in demonstrating the effectiveness of this ancient healing and rejuvenative science. It is also my hope that health-care around the world will move in its approach from mere management of symptoms to genuine cure of disease.

Conclusion

Panchakarma's five procedures offer the most effective treatments for cleansing the body and eliminating the root of disease. They remove the substances which weaken the body and break down health, and restore life to balance and wholeness. As a result, the mind, body and senses become much more receptive to the food, medicine and *rasayanas* or rejuvenative preparations they receive to maintain health. These five therapies represent the ultimate in *shodhana chikitsa*, "treatment that eliminates the cause of disease." In contrast, many medical systems offer only *shamana chikitsa*, the practice of palliating symptoms, rather than healing their cause.

As a word of caution, these procedures are very delicate and patient-specific in their application. It is better that *Panchakarma* therapy not be done at all than to be done incorrectly. Therefore, it should always be performed under the supervision of an Ayurvedic physician trained in the science of *Panchakarma*.

After finishing the major eliminative procedures, *Panchakarma* concludes with treatments designed to rebuild, nourish and strengthen the body, called *Paschatkarma*, or post-procedures. The importance of this final stage of *Panchakarma*, which we'll discuss in the next chapter, cannot be underestimated. The *dhatus* need to be nourished and, in some cases, reconstructed, and the digestive fires — the body's metabolic processes — must be brought back to full capacity. Remember that almost all disease results from weak or incomplete metabolism. When the *agnis* are strong, health is strong.

---

* I was invited by Dr. Cousens to conduct and supervise a study at his Center in Arizona on *Panchakarma* therapy protocols which I divised in India. Eighteen patients were selected and evaluated by Dr. Cousens to experience one week of *Panchakarma*. Two scientific instruments were used in the evaluation of each patient. One, was an electric device modeled on the Voll technology. It measures the drop in galvanic resistence in the meridians. The second instrument used was a darkfield microscope amplified with a Nassens condenser. The method of evaluation was the German system as outlined by Enderlin. Though these two instruments are not widely accepted in the U.S. scientific community, they are in Europe.

The above study was a preliminary one, though the initial results were extremely encouraging. We were able to demonstrate, with scientific instrumentation, that there is a significant positive change in the individuals health profile through the intervention of *Panchakarma*.

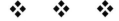

Chapter Eleven

PANCHAKARMA:
POST-TREATMENT PROCEDURES

anchakarma therapy can be likened to a surgical operation in which the pre-operative and post-operative procedures are of critical importance. Without the
preparatory procedures of *snehana* and *swedana*, internal cleansing
is superficial and does not remove the basis of disease. Once the
toxins and waste products are eliminated from the gastrointestinal
tract by *nasya*, *vamana*, *virechana* and *nirooha bastis*, both the digestive *agni* and the *dhatus* must have the opportunity to rebuild
themselves.

The set of procedures that follow the main eliminative treatments of *Panchakarma* and assist this rebuilding process are called,
collectively, *Paschatkarma*. They assure the re-establishment of
healthy metabolic function and immunity. If these post-procedures are neglected, digestion does not normalize. Weak digestion
generates new *ama* and the tissues continue to receive toxic material instead of nutritive, strengthening substances. The body then
finds it difficult to re-establish its natural immune function and is
more likely to fall ill again.

While the digestive fires are rekindling, it is important to
respect the somewhat vulnerable state of the physiology. Energy
resources are not at their full capacity and, as a result, we cannot
do as much as we will be able to do once the *dhatus* are rebuilt and
up to speed. It is therefore crucial for the success of *Panchakarma*
that the patient follow a regulated diet and lifestyle immediately
after treatment. Two aspects of the post-procedures — *samsara-*

jana krama and *dinacharya* —-- raise the system to a much higher efficiency level than it had before. A third aspect of *Paschatkarma*, called *rasayana* therapy, is not technically part of *Panchakarma*, but is particularly helpful in rejuvenating the *dhatus*.

SAMSARAJANA KRAMA: GRADUATED DIET

Digestion is the first aspect of the physiology that needs to be reconstructed. The *Panchakarma* treatments dramatically affect the digestive process because the G-I tract provides the primary route for the elimination of toxins. The digestive fire is weakened by the process of *ama* being drawn back into the digestive tract and expelled from the body.

Since faulty digestion creates the potential for illness to arise in the first place, special attention is given to strengthening digestion at the conclusion of *Panchakarma*. This assures that the *dhatus* are nourished, immunity is re-established, and health is maintained.

Samsarajana krama constitutes the primary post-treatment procedure for digestion. This term literally means "a graded administration of diet." It consists of a specially prepared diet designed to re-establish full digestive capacity and prevent the formation of new *ama*.

Charaka uses the following example to show the similarity between digestive *agni* and fire. If someone wants to kindle a fire that can consume a large quantity of dense wood, he must begin with a spark and some blades of dry grass. Once the grass is burning, small splinters and twigs can be added, then small branches and finally heavy logs. Once the logs are burning, the fire can consume any wood added to it. If, however, a log is added to the first spark and the few blades of burning grass, it extinguishes the fire.

In the same way, food is the fuel that ignites our activities. If, at the end of the main procedures, the food we ingest is too heavy for our exhausted digestive fires to manage, then little or none of that food will be metabolized and transformed into usable nutritive substances. It all becomes *ama* and the disease process starts anew. This is an unpleasant thought, but luckily it is a situation that is completely avoidable through correct administration of diet.

The diet given to the patient immediately after *Panchakarma* consists of nutritive and easily digested preparations of rice and split yellow mung *dal* (lentil). The diet is structured in stages, going from more liquid preparations to increasingly solid ones. It begins with easily digestible rice water, and eventually incorporates *dal*. These stages of digestibility are called *manda*, *peya*, *vilepi*, *odana*, *yusha* and *kichari*. Once this regimen has nurtured our digestive fire back to health, as signaled by a strong, consistent appetite, the person can return to a normal diet.

Manda: Rice Water

Manda, meaning "liquid," is the first meal after *vamana* or *virechana*. It is normally taken when the appetite returns, which for most people is about four hours after completing these procedures. *Manda* is mainly just the water in which *basmati* rice was boiled. It should be eaten lukewarm with a little *ghee* and a pinch of black salt (*saindhava*). It might seem absurd to give only rice water after these major procedures, but the importance of going slowly at this time, due to depleted digestive capacity, cannot be emphasized enough.

Peya: Rice Soup

The patient takes the next meal, called *peya*, two to three hours later. *Peya* means "soup" and is traditionally made with eight parts water to one part rice. The rice is cooked until it is very soft, so that it has the consistency of a thin, light porridge.

Vilepi: Thick Rice Soup

Vilepi, or "thick soup," describes the third and fourth meals after *vamana* or *virechana*. *Vilepi* consists of a slightly thicker porridge of soft, cooked rice grains and is made with a ratio of four parts water to one part grain. A little black salt and dried sugarcane juice can be added for taste. In order to add some strength to the digestive fire, one can lightly sauté a little fresh ginger, turmeric, cumin, coriander or fennel in a small amount of *ghee* and add them to the porridge. All these spices are high in *agni bhuta*.

Odana: Cooked Rice

Odana, which means "cooked rice" and has the consistency of normal, soft, cooked rice, is given as the fifth meal.

Yusha: Mung Lentil Soup

Dal is added to the sixth meal, which the patient eats on the second day after *virechana* and *vamana*. *Yusha*, or "soup mixture," is rice with some yellow mung *dal* (split, hulled mung lentils) added. It is important that each of these preparations should be made fresh daily.

Kichari: Rice and *Dal* Mixture

The patient now gets *kichari* for a number of meals. *Kichari* contains a mixture of *basmati* rice and split yellow mung *dal* cooked together with a pinch of black salt and the sautéed spices mentioned above. This nourishing food forms the basis of the traditional purification, recuperation and rejuvenation diets in *Panchakarma* therapy. It is easy to digest, provides complete and balanced nutrition, and is suitable for people with all types of constitutions since it balances all three *doshas*. It strengthens all the *dhatus* while assisting the detoxification process. (The recipe for *kichari* was provided in Chapter Nine, page 200).

The length of time it takes for patients to return to a normal diet depends on their digestive capacity. On the average, it takes six to seven meals. However, some people may only need three or four meals while others may require eight to ten. The Ayurvedic physician monitors the strength of the patient's digestive *agni* and adjusts the diet according to the strength of his appetite.

One of Ayurveda's strongest prescriptions is to eat only when hungry. This is doubly true of the time immediately following *Panchakarma*. The patient should only eat when his appetite is strong. A good appetite is our body's signal that digestion, assimilation and elimination are working well. One of the best ways to help quickly restore the appetite is to drink freshly grated, ginger root tea morning and afternoon.

Since proper digestion is essential to maintaining good health, it is important to maintain the strength of the digestive fires once they are up to full force. Ayurveda offers the following as some general guidelines for doing this. Some of these points have already been mentioned in previous chapters.

1. Only eat when you have an appetite.
2. Do not eat to full capacity. Always leave a little room in your stomach at the end of each meal.
3. Avoid drinking cold liquids with your meals.
4. Eat your main meal at noontime when the environmental *agni* is strongest, and eat a lighter meal at night.
5. Eat in a calm atmosphere and sit down when you eat.
6. When possible, avoid snacks between meals and avoid eating just before going to bed.
7. Once every week or two, fast or eat lightly to give your digestion a much needed rest.
8. Avoid foods that are deep-fried or too heavy.

DINACHARYA: GRADUATED LIFESTYLE

Along with a graduated diet, the post-procedures of *Panchakarma* prescribe gradations in lifestyle. In other words, the patient is strongly urged to move back into activity gradually, so that the delicate state of the nervous system is not over-taxed. The resources of the body must keep pace with the ability of the metabolic processes to supply it with energy, otherwise it begins to run at a deficit. In addition, the *dhatus* need time to rebuild themselves.

Unfortunately, the demands of our active modern lifestyle often run counter to our physiological and psychological requirements after *Panchakarma*. We want to jump off the treatment table, catch a plane and be back at work Monday morning, a new person. Life's demands seem to snatch our time and attention with the lightning speed of a slight-of-hand artist and leave us with little or nothing in return. Our tendency to drive ourselves and disregard our needs are, in many ways, what have led us into the disease process in the first place. This tendency may also cause us to underestimate the profound impact that *Panchakarma* has had on our minds and bodies and cause us to ignore the need to reintegrate slowly into activity.

For *Panchakarma* to be completely successful, we must adopt a graduated re-entry program that supports and enhances the changes that have already occurred. The lifestyle program that we adopt as a part of post-procedures, and to support good health once we're back in full swing, is called *dinacharya*, or daily routine.

Ayurveda strongly suggests that patients plan for some downtime after the main procedures are complete to insure that their progression into activity is not too fast. If the contrast between the deep rest of *Panchakarma* and the dynamic activity of working life is too sudden, the system may experience a shock. It's like coming out of deep sleep or meditation too quickly: we feel headachy, disoriented and perhaps a bit irritable.

It will take some time to completely assimilate the benefits of *Panchakarma* therapy, so until the patients' energy level is normal and stable for a while, they are advised to avoid undue mental and physical stress, including travel, strenuous exercise and sexual activity. Immediately following *Panchakarma*, it is also important to avoid excessive exposure to the elements; i.e., unusually hot, windy, cold or rainy weather conditions. Sunbathing and swimming in cold water are particularly not advised for at least a week following *Panchakarma*.

Applying these guidelines supports and enhances the effects of the preparatory and eliminative procedures and assists the body in concentrating its energy on complete rejuvenation. The behavioral recommendations presented in Chapter Six under *Dinacharya*, page 154-155, are extremely useful during this period and afterwards for creating and maintaining a new level of health.

RASAYANA: HERBAL AND MINERAL REJUVENATION THERAPY

As we mentioned earlier, *rasayana karma* does not technically belong to *Panchakarma* therapy, but forms its own system within Ayurvedic science. However, the *rasayana* therapy increases the effectiveness of *Panchakarma*'s rejuvenating processes. *Rasayana* actually means "that which increases the essence of each *dhatu*, starting with *rasa*."

When people hear about the rejuvenating properties of *rasayanas*, it is common for them to want to take them immediately, without going through the necessary procedures to make the body receptive to their influence. This will not work for three reasons:

(i) The *rasayanas* are very refined and concentrated herbal and mineral formulas that take a strong digestive capacity to metabolize.

(ii) Imbalanced *doshic* functioning impedes delivery of these substances to the *dhatus*.

(iii) The *ama* and *malas* stored in the *dhatus* block their ability to assimilate these special compounds.

As a result of these three factors, *rasayana* therapy does not generally achieve its desired effect until after *Panchakarma*. Digestion must be strengthened, the *doshas* must be balanced and impurities must be eliminated from the *dhatus* through *Panchakarma* therapy in order for the *rasayanas* to work.

The ancient texts prescribe many types of *rasayanas*, and each has a specific effect on body and mind. Some nourish the *dhatus*, reverse the effects of aging and re-enliven the body. Other formulas increase physical strength and stamina and help the immune system, as well as pacify and nourish the *doshas*. Certain *rasayanas*, like *vajikarana karma*, increase physical vitality, energy and virility and generate the reproductive health necessary to create healthy offspring. They also enhance spiritual vitality and mental strength.

Many herbs and herbal formulas are commonly given after *Panchakarma* to produce specific benefits:

- *Ashwagandha* pacifies and balances *vata*.

- *Brahmi* and *manjista* pacify *pitta*.

- Ginger, black pepper and *pippali* improve the digestive capacity of all the *dhatu agnis* and pacifies *kapha*.

- *Amalaki* increases *sattva*, thereby improving the clarity, stillness and positivity of the mind. It also pacifies both *pitta* and *vata*.

Most of the clinical experiences I have shared with you so far have related to the effectiveness of *Panchakarma* and *rasayana* therapies on specific diseased conditions. However, as I have repeatedly stated, Ayurveda and *Panchakarma* are ultimately about reestablishing a conscious connection to wholeness. The following case, and many like it, have repeatedly verified for me that this ancient system does, in fact, accomplish this goal.

A man came to me for *Panchakarma* therapy who had no real health problems of any consequence. Rather, his stated objective was to raise his level of awareness of the *atma* within himself. He underwent a six week program of cleansing and rejuvenation with *Panchakarma* and then I started him on a course of *rasayanas*. He subsequently related to me that about a month after completing the treatment, he experienced the dawning of a whole new level of awareness. He noticed his mental clarity and comprehension were much greater than they had ever been in the past. He also said that his sense of humor had grown to "outrageous proportions." But the most impressive result, he said, was the growth of a sense of lightness, freedom and non-attachment. He reported that he felt much more surrendered to the experience of the divine within himself, and that much of the "struggle of life" had dropped away.

Such an experience demonstrates that when the false covering of ill-health is removed from the mind, senses and body, our true nature or *prakruti* shines through and is intimately connected to the universal *prakruti*.

Expectations Surrounding *Panchakarma*

It is important to address the issue of what one can expect from this therapy. While *Panchakarma* alleviates symptoms of disease, its real objective is to eliminate their cause. In itself, the absence of symptoms does not always indicate a complete cure. Symptoms can often be quickly eliminated, but cure usually takes more time.

If a person has been storing the seeds of degenerative disease in his body for fifteen or twenty years and suffering from symptoms for five or ten years, it is unlikely that they will be completely healed in ten or fifteen days of *Panchakarma*. It takes time and repeated treatments to rid the body completely of *ama* and to rebuild and rejuvenate the *dhatus*. The length of the treatment varies with the type of illness and the adverse effects created by previous treatment procedures. Individuals also respond differently to *Panchakarma* treatment because of differences in their individual constitutions.

PANCHAKARMA REGIMENS

In his elaboration of the science of rejuvenation, *Charaka* prescribed the following *Panchakarma* regimen:

First Cycle
Seven days of *snehana*, *swedana* and *nasya*
Eighth day: *vamana*
Three days of *samarajana krama* after *vamana*

Second Cycle
Seven days of *snehana*, *swedana* and *nasya*
Eighth day: *virechana*
Three days of *samarajana krama* after *virechana*

Third Cycle
Eight, fifteen or thirty days of *snehana*, *swedana*, *nasya* and *basti* therapy, depending on the nature and severity of the illness. *Nasya* treatment can be performed separately from *basti*, but is still combined with *snehana* and *swedana*.

Sushruta Samhita confirms the effectiveness of the *Panchakarma* regimen, and in addition adds *raktamokshana*.

Though *Charaka* has provided this schedule as a general framework for the administration of *Panchakarma*, he categorically states that the Ayurvedic physician should use his own knowledge and expertise to design a treatment regimen which is appropriate for the patient and his or her illness.

Based on more than fifteen years of clinical experience and over 9,000 *Panchakarma* protocols, I have found the following month-long program to be very effective:

Days 1-7:	*Snehana, swedana, nasya* (cleansing) and *basti* (various combinations of *nirooha* and *anuwasan*)
Day 8:	*Vamana*
Days 9-10:	*Samsarajana krama* and rest
Days 11-15:	*Snehana, swedana, nasya* (cleansing) and *basti* (same as above)
Day 16:	*Virechana*
Days 17-18:	*Samsarajana krama* and rest
Days 19-26:	*Snehana, swedana, nasya* (nourishing) and *basti* (*bruhan* and *anuwasan*)
Days 27-28:	*Samsarajana krama* and rest

As you can tell, a strong emphasis is placed on *nasya* and *basti karma* to cleanse the body and to pacify and nourish *vata*; as we have mentioned so often in this book, *vata* is the prime mover of all functions in the body. When we control *vata*, we control health.

The whole treatment takes twenty-eight days, but I generally advise my patients to set aside a few days before and after the treatment program for reasons described above.

In the West, however, few people seem able to take this much time away from their work and responsibilities, so one-and two-week programs have been tailored. These abbreviated programs focus mainly on pacifying and nourishing *vata* and helping cleanse *ama* and *mala* from the *pitta* and *vata* zones of the body.

In this regimen, the preparatory procedures of *snehana* and *swedana* must be given for a minimum of seven days before administering *virechana*. This insures that all seven *dhatus* are completely oleated. During this seven day period, there is extensive use of *shodhana* or cleansing *nasyas* and *bastis*.

This one-week or two-week program is highly recommended once or twice a year for preventative purposes. It is even more beneficial when it can be performed around the change of seasons since this is the time when the *doshas* can most easily become imbalanced in their functioning. However, in cases of chronic or degenerative diseases, a longer-term treatment of at least one month is highly recommended. Depending on the seriousness and duration of the disorder, a series of such longer treatment programs may be necessary to remove the basis of the disease.

It is not always possible to take time away from one's family and profession to engage in *Panchakarma* therapy, even if we are in need of it. The next chapter offers some simple *shamana* (palliative) and *shodhana* (cleansing) procedures that you can do yourself when imbalances arise.

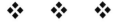

Chapter Twelve

SELF-CARE AT HOME

*A*ll the classical Ayurvedic texts emphasize the importance of receiving *Panchakarma* treatments under the supervision of physicians who are fully trained in *Panchakarma* therapy. During *Panchakarma*, the physician must monitor the patient's condition and responses and adjust the treatments accordingly, as well as support the patient in this process. The patient cannot make these detailed evaluations by himself. It is unfortunate that so few qualified Ayurvedic physicians exist in the West. Even in India, only a small number of Ayurvedic physicians have studied *Panchakarma* in depth and made it their specialty.

The practice of Ayurvedic medicine requires training and licensing procedures similar to those required of medical doctors in the United States. After the applicant meets certain prerequisites, he attends Ayurvedic medical college for five-and-a-half years and then takes an internship and vigorous licensing examinations. New Ayurvedic physicians then have the option to continue their training and consider *Panchakarma* as a specialty. This entails another three years of education and research and is equivalent to a Ph.D.

Fortunately, more and more young physicians are recognizing *Panchakarma*'s profound curative benefits and are choosing it over other specialties that favor more palliative approaches to treatment. While many patients still seek simple, quick methods to eliminate symptoms, increasing numbers of doctors are discovering the deep satisfaction that comes from removing the causes of illness and educating patients for health-maintenance once health is restored.

The amount of people researching and experiencing *Panchakarma* is also growing. After learning about *Panchakarma*, many individuals wish to use it not only to treat current disorders, but also to sustain health and happiness and prevent future disease.

Though you cannot administer full *Panchakarma* regimens safely and effectively to yourself, there are some treatments that can be done at home to help eliminate *ama* and *mala* from the body. Though these are technically not considered *Panchakarma* procedures and do not provide the comprehensive benefits of *Panchakarma* therapy, they are *shodhana*, or cleansing in nature, and have a definite preventive value.

Before you undertake *shodhana* self-care, you must have some understanding of your *vikruti*, or *doshic* imbalance. When you know this, you can adopt supportive dietary and lifestyle regimens and use some of the appropriate *shodhana* procedures.

Treating *Doshic* Imbalances

The test in Chapter Five, pages 115-119, will give you a rough understanding of your *vikruti*. In addition to this, note the condition of your appetite, digestion and elimination. Since all three *doshas* operate in the digestive tract, you will gain valuable clues as to where your imbalances lie.

If your appetite is frequently weak, your digestion is sluggish, you feel heavy and sleepy after eating and have excessive mucous secretions, sneezing and allergies, *kapha* is probably excessive. If you experience acidity, gas, bloating, sour burping, great thirst after eating or inner heat, it probably indicates *pitta* aggravation. If you have sluggish elimination, hard stools and frequent constipation; or if you feel extremely dry or cold and suffer from insomnia, anxiety or depression, then *vata dosha* is either excessive or obstructed. When you have *doshic* imbalances, your energy level is low or variable. While the following suggestions will not completely detoxify the body, they may reduce your symptoms and help you feel better.

TREATMENTS FOR *KAPHA* ZONE IMBALANCES

If you suffer from a *kapha* imbalance, Ayurveda recommends taking only vegetable juices for a few days. Make the juices fresh and use vegetables with a bitter and pungent taste, such as asparagus, beet greens, bitter melons, broccoli, cabbage, carrots, cauliflower, kale and leafy greens.

Sinus Congestion

If you experience congested sinuses or severe sinus headaches, then you can try cleansing the sinuses with the following nose drops. Take two drops of juice extracted from fresh ginger root; add one drop of fresh lime juice and half a pinch of *jaggery* or Sucanat (dried sugarcane juice). Mix well with a little warm water and put one drop in each nostril twice a day. Before administering the drops, gently massage your face and sinus area vigorously with a little warm sesame oil and apply a hot towel or hot water bottle to the sinus area.

Lie on your back with your head hanging off the end of the bed and place the drops in each nostril with the help of a dropper. Immediately afterwards, pinch the nostrils repeatedly while sniffing slowly and deeply. This helps draw the mixture up into the sinuses. Then again place a hot towel or hot water bottle over your nose and sinus area for a few minutes. You may experience a slight burning sensation as the drops are drawn up into the sinuses and then an increase in nasal secretions.

If you have a lot of burning in your nose, apply a little *ghee* to the inside of your nose. After you blow your nose, your nasal passages and head will generally feel clearer and lighter. After a few treatments, your symptoms should be reduced or gone. This procedure, however, is usually not recommended for those with *pitta* aggravation.

Daily Sinus Cleansing

Since the sinuses are the gateway to the brain, it is important to keep them clear and free of mucus so the flow of *prana* to this region remains unobstructed. The following cleansing stimuli can be used on a day-to-day basis to keep the sinuses open.

To sixteen ounces of water, add a half-inch of grated ginger, one teaspoon of licorice powder, one-quarter teaspoon of *pippali* and one-quarter teaspoon of *vacha*. Boil this solution until it is approximately four ounces, or one-quarter its original volume. To this add four ounces of sesame oil and boil until the remaining water is evaporated. Strain the contents and store the oil in a sterile, airtight dropper bottle.

To administer the solution, lie on your back with your head off the end of the bed, or simply tilt your head back while in a standing position and place two drops in each nostril. Then pinch your nostrils repeatedly while inhaling deeply through the nose. It is important to warm the oil before each application. You can do this by placing the dropper bottle in hot water for a few minutes. Though this procedure is particularly effective in the early morning, you can also use it when needed during the day.

Sore Throat

For a sore or inflamed throat, mix a little powdered turmeric and uncooked honey together in a paste and take one-half teaspoon of this preparation three times a day. This should reduce the inflammation.

Throat Congestion

If you experience uncomfortable amounts of mucus in your throat and larynx in the early mornings, prepare a warm saline solution with a pinch of turmeric, and gargle.

Early Morning Nausea

When you wake up in the morning, if you have sweet, sticky, watery secretions in your mouth, or experience nausea and the urge to throw up, you have accumulated excess *kapha*, as well as mucus in the stomach and *kapha* zone. To counteract this condition, first thing in the morning, on an empty stomach, drink one liter (approximately one quart) of fresh warm licorice root tea. This may make you feel a little warm and nauseous. Now induce vomiting by tickling the inside of your throat with your finger. By patiently expelling all of the licorice tea, you will also bring up the accumulated mucus and cleanse your esophagus and stomach. Afterwards you can drink a little warm water. After about two hours, you can eat a meal of light, easily digestible soup.

This technique should not be confused with *vamana*, *Panchakarma*'s major eliminative procedure to purify the *kapha* zone. It does, however, quickly cleanse excess *kapha* and toxins from the stomach and alleviate the symptoms. This should only be used in the case of acute symptoms and should never be attempted if you have esophageal disorders, diverticulitis, gastric ulcers or hiatal hernia.

Colds and Congestion

To reduce abundant *kapha*, you can drink *kapha* tea and follow a *kapha*-pacifying diet and lifestyle. If you have symptoms of cold, cough, congestion or flu, you can drink ginger and turmeric tea every four hours. You can also take one-quarter teaspoon of *pippali* powder with honey three times a day until your symptoms disappear. For nasal congestion, inhale the steam from eucalyptus oil, which dissolves blocks in the sinuses.

TREATMENTS FOR *PITTA* ZONE IMBALANCES

To counteract symptoms associated with excess *pitta*, Ayurveda advises refraining from food and drink with pungent, sour and salty tastes, such as fermented, deep-fried or hot, spicy foods. It also strongly recommends that you avoid stressful and aggravating situations.

General *Pitta* Disorders

The following simple procedure helps to remove some of the *pitta*-related *ama* and calm down excess *pitta*. You should use this technique on a day that you don't have to work and can stay relaxed.

On the evening before treatment, make some fresh ginger-root tea by boiling one or two inches of grated or finely sliced ginger-root in one cup of water. Boil the tea to about three-quarters of a cup, strain out the ginger and add twenty milliliters (four teaspoons) of castor oil. Mix it well and drink it when the evening *pitta* cycle begins, around 10 P.M. The next morning some purging will take place which will help to cleanse the *pitta* zone. Take it easy for the rest of the day and eat only soups or *kichari* if you feel hungry.

Hyperacidity

Pitta tea and a *pitta*-pacifying diet and lifestyle all help reduce excess *pitta*. Pomegranate juice also works well. If you have problems with too much heat and acidity, you can take a tablespoon each of licorice-root powder and turmeric root powder, three times a day in between meals.

If you are experiencing burning when you urinate or defecate, then you can make a tea with one teaspoon each of fennel, cumin and coriander seeds in two cups of water. Boil it down to one cup and sip during the day. Do this for two to three days.

Skin Rashes

If you are suffering from mild skin rashes, massage with coconut oil and drink the same tea recommended above.

Menopause

Women who are entering menopause often suffer from hot flashes, night sweats and irritability. In addition to a *pitta*-pacifying diet and lifestyle, you can use one-teaspoon each of *ashwagandha, shatavari and amalaki,* taken between meals twice a day for at least three months.

PMS: Premenstrual Syndrome

PMS, a common discomfort plaguing many women, is, according to Ayurveda, caused by an accumulation of *ama* which blocks the *shrotas*. In the days immediately before and during the menstrual cycle, drink warm water upon arising and sip ginger tea throughout the day. Make this tea with fresh ginger-root, fennel seeds, licorice powder and cumin powder. Avoid salt, sugar and fermented foods, and in the evening, before dinner, chew well a tablespoon each of sesame seeds and organic raisins to improve elimination. It is also important to perform both *abhyanga* (described below in the section on treating *vata* imbalances) in the morning to improve circulation and *pranayama* to improve the flow of *prana* in the body. It is also strongly recommended to meditate daily to reduce the mental agitation that often comes with this condition.

TREATMENTS FOR *VATA* ZONE IMBALANCES

For symptoms related to excess *vata*, Ayurveda recommends following a *vata*-pacifying diet and lifestyle. In particular, avoid cold, windy conditions, too much stress, exercise and travel, and foods that are hard, rough, dry and cold.

General *Vata* Disorders

One of the best procedures for conditions involving *vata* aggravation is *abhyanga* , a daily self-administered oil massage. This treatment is most successful in pacifying *vata* when it is done early in the morning or late in the afternoon, the times when *vayu* dominates the environment and *vata* dominates the physiology. Use sesame oil that has been cured, or heated to about 180 degrees and then allowed to cool to just above body temperature. Curing the oil in this manner makes it easier for the body to assimilate.

You can prepare approximately one pint of oil at a time and use it over the following few days. Use caution in curing oil, since it is flammable. It should never be left unattended. In order to determine if the sesame oil has reached the right temperature for curing, put a drop of water in the oil. If the water sputters on the surface, the oil is properly cured.

Warm a small amount of the cured oil each day to just above body temperature by placing a small plastic bottle of the oil in a sink full of hot water for a few minutes. Massage the oil into your skin using straight, long strokes over the long areas of the body (arms, legs, sides and back) and circular strokes over the joints. Start with the head and upper part of the body and proceed downwards to the feet.

During *abhyanga*, a little extra attention should be given to the face, the crown of the head, the ears and the soles of the feet. After massaging oil into the whole body, soak in a warm bath or shower to open the *shrotas*. It's beneficial to leave a small amount of oil on to nourish and protect the skin. To facilitate this, use little or no soap after soaking and simply towel off any excess oil.

Dry Nasal Passages

Prati marshya nasya helps *vata* conditions involving dryness in the nasal and sinus passages. Put a small amount of *ghee* or sesame oil (preferably warm) into your nose several times a day, gently massaging the inside of each nostril. This helps protect you from the *vata*-aggravating influence of dry, windy or cold weather, as well as airborne allergens and pollutants.

Irregularity

Ayurveda recommends *matra bastis* when you have incomplete elimination or when travel's *vata*-aggravating effects make you feel unsettled. To prepare the *basti*, soak one tablespoon of *dashmoola* (a standard Ayurvedic mixture consisting of ten herbal roots) overnight (approximately ten to twelve hours) in 400 milliliters (approximately one-and-three-quarters cups) of pure water. Boil the mixture for ten to fifteen minutes until the volume is reduced to three-quarters of the original volume, or approximately 300 milliliters. Strain the water and add thirty milliliters (two tablespoons) of sesame oil, one half teaspoon uncooked honey and a pinch (approximately one-sixteenth of a teaspoon) of black salt (*saindhava* or *kala namak*). Mix or shake the mixture well until the oil and water are well homogenized.

Administer this *basti* fluid using an enema bag or a large plastic syringe with a rubber catheter attached, see page 243, (available at medical supply stores). The *basti* fluid should be warm but not hot. The best time for the *basti* is late afternoon or early evening, the *vata*-dominant times of day. Introduce the *basti* into the rectum slowly and, if possible, retain it in the body for at least forty-five minutes. These *bastis* successfully diminish and settle *vata* and improve colon function.

Diet and lifestyle constitute key factors in the successful management of *vata*. The following daily practices significantly help with *vata* pacification.

1. Avoid stress and strain as much as possible.

2. Do *abhyanga* massage with warm sesame oil, followed by a hot bath or shower, in the early morning or late afternoon.

3. Apply a little *ghee* or oil to the inside of the nostrils several times daily.

4. Practice *asanas* or Hatha Yoga postures, especially the locust, cobra and knee-to-chest positions.

5. Practice *pranayama*, alternate nostril breathing, for several minutes, preferably before meditation.

6. Practice a relaxing form of meditation that brings stillness and silence to the mind and senses.

7. Do not over-exercise.

8. Drink *vata* tea and eat a *vata*-reducing diet, avoiding dry, porous, hard, rough or leftover foods. Eat naturally sweet, warm, slightly oily or fatty foods and follow a relaxed and regular daily routine.

Conclusion

In the 20th century, mankind has significantly altered the quality of the basic ingredients to survival, i.e., air, water, earth, and food. As a result, the very existence of the species is now threatened in a significant way. We are part and parcel of nature, at whose core are the five basic elements — space, air, fire, water, earth. When we learn to live in alignment with the laws and cycles of nature, nature supports health and well-being. Through this connection with nature and the power of radiant health, we bring joy to others and balance and progress to society. Ayurveda always seeks to remind people that this is their birthright and responsibility.

If we are to survive into the 21st century, we must address the damage we have inflicted upon Mother Nature in polluting our air, water, earth and food. This is our only hope if we expect the quality of our lives to improve. More importantly, will we make the choice to survive as a species?

Health lies within the reach of all of us. Ayurveda wishes everyone to enjoy the happiness, productivity and satisfaction that comes with good health. I hope this book has assisted you on your journey to perfect health, longevity and enlightenment.

Shubham bhavatu! God bless you!

BIBLIOGRAPHY

Ashtanga Hrudaya (Bhagirathi Tippanni), translated by Pundit Taradutta Panta, Jaikrishnadas Haridas Gupta, Chaukhambha, Varanasi, India, 1939

Ashtanga-Sangraha, translated by Atridev Vidyalanker, Volumes I, II, III & IV, Banaras Hindu University, Varanasi, India, 1962

Chakrapani Dutta (Tika) History of Ayurveda by Prof. P.V. Sharma, Chaukhambha Orientela, Varanasi, India, 1981

Charaka Samhita, translated by Pundit Krushna Shastri & Dr. Gorakhanath Chaturvedi, Volumes I & II, Choukambha Vishwabharati, Varanasi, India, 1982

Madhava Nidan, by Sudarshan Shastri, Volumes I & II, Choukambha Vishwabharati, Varanasi, India, 1981

Panchakarma Chikitsa Therapy, by Vaidya Haridas Shridhar Kasture, Shri Baidyanath Ayurved Bhavan Ltd, Nagpur, India, 1979

Sharirkriya Vigyan, by Prof. B.V. Sathye, Poona University, Pune, India, 1974

Sushruta Samhita, translated by Kaviraj Ambika dutta Shastri, Volumes I & II, Chaukhambha Vishwabharati, Varanasi, India, 1982

Vyadhi-Vinischayua, by Vaidya A.D. Athawale and Vaidya Nirmala Raywade and Vaidya S.A. Joshi, Madhav D. Gurjar-Ayurvidya Mudranalaya, Pune, India, 1984

GLOSSARY

Abhyanga: Daily oil massage to increase circulation, decrease dryness and reduce *vata* aggravation.

Abhyantar Snehana: Internal oleation. Part of *Purvakarma* (the preparatory procedures of *Panchakarma*), it is specifically designed to liquefy and dislodge *ama* from the *dhatus*.

Agni: The element and universal organizing principle of conversion, light and heat.

Agni Swedana: A procedure used to promote sweating and dilation of channels through heating the body.

Ahara: The Ayurvedic knowledge of proper diet. One of the three pillars of Ayurveda.

Akash: The element and universal organizing principle of space.

Alochak Pitta: The metabolic function associated with the eye.

Ama: The toxic residue of undigested food that is the source of illness in the body.

Anuloman: The aspect of gastrointestinal vitality concerned with proper elimination.

Anuwasan Basti: An oil *basti* which is meant to be retained in the colon for a long period of time.

Apana Vayu: The sub-*dosha* of *vata* which governs the elimination of waste.

Asanas: Hatha yoga postures designed to refine physiological functioning.

Asatmya-Indriyartha-Samyog: The improper uses of the senses.

Asthi: The *dhatu* or bodily tissue of bone.

Atma: The universal intelligence of nature. Also known as *param atma*.

Aushadhi: The Ayurvedic management of disease. One of the three pillars of Ayurveda.

Avapidana Nasya: Herbal mixtures crushed and squeezed into the nostrils.

Ayurveda: The science of life, the oldest health-care science known to man.

Bahya Snehana: External oleation used during *Purvakarma* (the preparatory procedures of *Panchakarma*), specifically designed to liquefy and dislodge *ama* from the *dhatus*.

Bashpa Swedana: Steam bath. Part of the preparatory procedures of *Panchakarma* specifically used to dilate the *shrotas* or channels of the body to facilitate the removal of *ama*.

Basti: Therapeutic purification and rejuvenation of the colon. One of the five main procedures of *Panchakarma*.

Bheda: The sixth stage of disease manifestation characterized by complications.

Bhrajak Pitta: The metabolic function associated with the skin.

Bhutas: The five elements.

Bruhan Nasya: Medicated oil introduced into the nostrils to nourish both the senses and the brain.

Chandan Bala Oil: Medicated oil used in *bahya snehana* to pacify *pitta dosha*.

Charaka: The original commentator on Ayurveda, considered to be the father of Ayurveda.

Charaka Samhita: The first and most authoritative commentary on Ayurveda.

Dal: Split yellow mung lentil soup.

Deepan: The aspect of gastrointestinal vitality concerned with promoting strong digestive fire.

Dharma: Lifes purpose.

Dhatu Agni: The metabolic function associated with each of the seven *dhatus*.

Dhatus: The seven retainable substances or structures of the body. Bodily tissues.

Dhi: Intellect. The aspect of *sattva* that imparts the ability to conceive and imagine.

Dhruti: The positive aspect of *rajas* that imparts the ability to implement creative thought.

Dinacharya: Daily behavioral guidelines for maintaining ideal health.

Dosha: The functional intelligence within the human body responsible for all physiological and psychological processes.

Dosha Gati: The twice daily movement that each *dosha* follows from the hollow structures of the gastrointestinal tract to the thicker structures of the *dhatus* and back again. Also the movement of the *doshas* from their seats in the G-I tract to their nearest orifice.

Drava Swedana: The use of hot baths to promote sweating.

Dwandaj: A condition where two *doshas* have an equally dominant influence in a persons *prakruti* or constitutional make-up.

Gandush: Gargling with a warm saline solution.

Gati: Mobility

Ghee: Clarified butter.

Gunas: The three phases of activity in creation as well as the three qualities of the mind.

Indriyas: The five senses. One of the four components of Ayu.

Jaggery: Dried, unprocessed sugarcane juice.

Jala: The element and universal organizing principle of liquidity and cohesion. Also known as the water element.

Jathara Agni: The digestive fire, located in the gastrointestinal tract.

Jiva Atma: The individual soul. One of the four components of Ayu.

Kal Basti: A *basti* that is administered at a specific time for maximum effect.

Kapha: The *dosha* or functional intelligence within the body governing cohesion, liquidity and growth.

Kapikachhu: An herb used to improve the function of *shukra dhatu*.

Karma: An action or procedure used in *Panchakarma* therapy.

Karma Basti: A month-long *basti* regimen administered to treat *vata*-related disorders.

Katti Basti: An external, localized application of medicated oil used in the region of the back.

Kaya Kalpa: Ancient rejuvenation procedure.

Kichari: A mixture of *basmati* rice and split yellow mung *dal* used to cleanse and balance the *doshas* during *Panchakarma* therapy.

Ksheer Basti: A medicated milk decoction administered through the rectum which nourishes all the *dhatus* of the body.

Lekhana Basti: A strong, penetrating, cleansing *basti*, used specifically to reduce *kapha dosha* and *meda dhatu*.

Lichen planus syndrome: A skin disease.

Mahabhutas: The universal organizing principles which structure and govern all physical phenomena.

Mahanarayana Oil: A medicated oil used in *bahya snehana* (the external oleation procedures of *Purvakarma*) specifically to pacify *kapha dosha*.

Majja: The *dhatu* or bodily tissue of bone marrow. Also, the term used to describe the bone marrow fat used on occasion in *abyantar snehana* (internal oleation).

Mala: The natural metabolic by-products which are always eliminated from the body.

Mamsa: The *dhatu* or bodily tissue of muscle.

Manas: The mind. One of the four components of *Ayu*.

Manda: Rice water. The first meal eaten after *Panchakarma*.

Marma: Sensitive points which represent a greater concentration of the body's vital force in that area.

Marsha Nasya: Repeated introduction of medicated oil into the nostrils used to clean, lubricate and strengthen the mucous membranes.

Matra Basti: A small self-administered oil *basti* that can be used at any time of the day, most commonly used to reduce the *vata*-aggravating effects of travel, exercise and stress.

Meda: The *dhatu* or bodily tissue of fat (adipose tissue).

Nadis: Very fine *shrotas* or channels of the body.

Nadi Swedana: Localized, penetrating steam administered specifically to the joints and spinal area during *Purvakarma* .

Nasya: The therapeutic cleansing of the head and neck region. One of the five purificatory procedures of *Panchakarma*.

Netra Basti: An external, localized application of medicated *ghee* around the eyes used to nourish the eyes, reduce eye strain and improve vision.

Netra Tarpana: Same as *Netra Basti*.

Nirooha Basti: A large, herbalized decoction administered into the colon to remove toxins and wastes from the body.

Ojakshaya: Depletion of *ojas*.

Ojas: the most refined product of *dhatu* metabolism which controls the body's immune function.

Pachak Pitta: The metabolic function occurring in the small intestine.

Pachan: The aspect of gastrointestinal vitality concerned with improving digestion and metabolism.

Pakwashaya Gata Basti: *Basti* administered through the rectum. The main type of *basti* used in *Panchakarma*.

Panchakarma: The five major purificatory procedures and adjunct therapies for purifying and rejuvenating the body.

Panchamahabhuta: The theory of the five elements.

Panchendriya Vardhan Oil: Oil used in *nasya* to nourish sensory functioning.

Param Atma: The universal intelligence of nature.

Parinam: The negative effects of the seasons on the body. The third major cause of disease after *pragya aparadha* and *astmya-indriyartha-samyog*.

Paryushit: Food that no longer contains vital force or *prana*

Paschatkarma: The post-procedures of *Panchakarma* therapy.

Peya: Rice soup. The second meal eaten after the main procedures of *Panchakarma* have been administered.

Pinda Swedana: A fomentation procedure performed with a bolus of rice and a hot milk decoction to tonify the muscles and improve the circulation

Pishinchhali: A vigorous herbal massage using a bolus of rice and a large amount of oil to improve the mobility of muscles and ligaments.

Pitta: The *dosha* or functional intelligence within the body governing all metabolic processes.

Pragya aparadha: The mistake of the intellect. Considered by Ayurveda to be the foremost cause of disease.

Prakopa: The second stage of disease manifestation characterized by provocation or aggravation of *ama* at its site of origin (in the G-I tract).

Prakruti: The inherent balance of *doshas* that is most beneficial to one's life. The constitution we are born with.

Prana: life-force or vital force.

Prana Vayu: The sub-*dosha* of *Vata* which governs sensory functions and the intake of *prana*, water and food.

Pranayama: An alternate nostril breathing exercise which increases the intake of *prana*. One of the three exercises of *vyayama*.

Prapaka Metabolism: The three transient phases of digestion that take place in the gastrointestinal tract.

Prasara: The third stage of disease manifestation characterized by the migration of *ama* from its site of origin (in the G-I tract).

Prati Marsha Nasya: Repeated application of medicated oil to the nostrils with the tip of the little finger to soothe dry mucous membranes and to protect against airborne allergens.

Prithvi: The element and universal organizing principle of form and structure. Also commonly known as the earth element.

Purvakarma: The set of procedures used to prepare a person for the main purificatory procedures of *Panchakarma*.

Rajas: The active phase of the mind. It imparts motivation and initiative to the mind. Also one of the three *guna*s or phases of activity in creation.

*Rajas*ic: Pertaining to the qualities of *rajas*.

Rakta: The *dhatu* or bodily tissue of blood.

Raktamokshana: Therapeutic withdrawal of blood. One of the five major purificatory procedures of *Panchakarma*.

Ranjak Pitta: The metabolic function associated with the liver.

Rasa: The *dhatu* or bodily tissue of plasma or nutrient-fluid. Also refers to the three categories of taste.

Rasayana: One of the branches of Ayurvedic science having to do with rejuvenation.

Rasayana Basti: A type of *basti* which has a rejuvenative influence on all the *dhatus*.

Rutucharya: The diet and lifestyle regimen prescribed by *vihara* to take into account the impact of each of the seasons on the body.

Sadhak Pitta: The metabolic function which controls the neuropeptides in the brain as well as mental processes.

Saindhava: Black salt

Samana Vayu: The sub-*dosha* of *vata* which governs the metabolism and distribution of nutrients in the body.

Samsarajana krama: The graded administration of diet. One of the post-procedures of *Panchakarma* concerned with strengthening the debilitated digestive fire.

Sanchaya: The first stage of disease manifestation characterized by the accumulation of *ama* in the gastrointestinal tract.

Sattva: The creative phase of the mind. The quality that imparts curiosity, inspiration and creativity to the mind. One of the three *guna*s or phases of activity in creation.

Sattvic: Pertaining to the qualities of *sattva*.

Shamana Basti: A therapeutic administration of medicated oil or decoction through the rectum to reduce irritation in the colon.

Shamana Chikitsa: One of the two primary methods of disease management whose purpose is only to palliate the symptoms of disease.

Shamana Nasya: A therapeutic administration of herbalized oil into the nostrils to soothe the sinus zone.

Sharira: The human body. One of the four components of *Ayu*.

Shat Kriya Kal: The six stages of disease manifestation.

Shiro Basti: Medicated oil administered to head which improves *prana* and sensory functioning.

Shirodhara: One of the adjunct procedures of *Purvakarma* designed to calm the mind and pacify *vata* in the central nervous system.

Shirovirechana: Therapeutic cleansing of head and neck region. Also called *Nasya*, it is one of the five main purificatory procedures of *Panchakarma*.

Shodhana Basti: A therapeutic administration of medicated decoctions to cleanse the colon of toxic substances and waste products.

Shodhana Chikitsa: One of the two primary methods of disease management whose focus is to eliminate the source of disease.

Shodhana Nasya: A therapeutic administration of medicated oil into the nostrils to eliminate toxins from the paranasal sinus zone.

Shrotas: The gross and subtle channels of the body.

Shukra: The male and female reproductive tissue of the body.

Smriti: Memory. More specifically, the positive aspect of *tamas* that imparts the ability to remember those things that are beneficial for our lives.

Sthana Samshraya: The fourth stage of disease manifestation characterized by augmentation of the disease process.

Surya Namaskar: Sun salutation in *Hatha Yoga asanas*.

Sushruta: One of the main commentators of Ayurvedic science after *Charaka*, whose focus was surgical procedures and purification of the blood.

Sushruta Samhita: *Sushruta* commentary on Ayurveda.

Swedana: One of the two main *Purvakarmas* (preparatory procedures of *Panchakarma*) whose purpose is to dilate the channels of the body so that the *doshas* can easily transport the dislodged *ama* back to the G-I tract for elimination.

Taila: Oil.

Tamas: The phase in the mind that brings activity to an end. It imparts dullness and inertia to the mind and causes a loss of knowingness. One of the three *guna*s or phase of activity in creation.

Tamasic: Pertaining to the quality of *tamas*.

Tapa Swedana: The application of dry heat to the body to reduce inflammation and congestion in the joints.

Tikta Ghrita: Medicated *ghee* with a predominantly bitter taste used in *abyantar snehana* (internal oleation) to remove *ama* from the *dhatus*.

Til Oil: Sesame oil.

Triphala: A laxative, combination of three fruits.

Udana Vayu: One of the sub-*doshas* of *vayu* which governs strength, speech and the elimination of carbon dioxide.

Udvartana: A type of therapeutic massage using powder instead of oil to reduce *meda dhatu* and excess *kapha*.

Upanaha Swedana: A therapeutic application of warm, medicated poultices used to treat arthritis.

Uro Basti: Medicated oils that are retained on the chest and heart area to reduce congestion.

Utkleshana Basti: Therapeutic administration of medicated decoctions through the rectum to promote secretions in the colon which liquefy and expel *ama* and waste material.

Vagabhata: A major commentator on Ayurvedic science after *Charaka* and *Sushruta*.

Vaidya: An Ayurvedic physician.

Vaishamya: The proportionate influence of the *doshas* that allows us to perceive the predominance of one over the others.

Vajirarana Basti: A *basti* which promotes vigor and vitality. Also used to enhance fertility.

Vamana: Therapeutic vomiting or emesis. One of the five main purificatory procedures of *Panchakarma*.

Vasa: An oleated substance composed of animal fat used in *abhyantar snehana* (internal oleation).

Vata: The *dosha* or functional intelligence in the body that governs movement, transportation and the drying and separating functions.

Vata Shamak Oil: The medicated oil used in *bahya snehana* (one of the main procedures of *Purvakarma*) to pacify *vata*.

Vayu: The element and universal organizing principle of movement. Also commonly known as the air or wind element.

Veda: The knowledge of the totality of life.

Vihara: The Ayurvedic knowledge of proper lifestyle. One of the three pillars of Ayurveda.

Vikruti: The imbalance in the *doshas* that obscures ones *prakruti* or ideal constitutional balance.

Vilepi: Thick soup of soft cooked rice usually eaten on the second day after *Panchakarma*.

Vipaka: The post-absorptive phase of digestion.

Virechana: Therapeutic purgation. One of the five main purificatory procedures of *Panchakarma*.

Vranagata Basti: Medicated liquids used to irrigate and heal abscesses or wounds.

Vyakta: The fifth stage of disease manifestation characterized by the manifestation of a clear set of symptoms.

Vyana Vayu: One of the sub-*doshas* of *Vata* which governs the cardiovascular system.

Vyayama: Three exercises prescribed by *vihara* which give energy rather than expend energy: *hatha yoga* postures, *pranayama* and sun salutation.

Yog Basti: An eight-day oil *basti* regimen specifically designed to calm *vata* and nourish the colon.

Yusha: Dal (yellow mung lentil soup) eaten on the second day after *Panchakarma*.

RESOURCES

Training in Ayurvedic Lifestyle Counseling and Pancha-karma is offered by Drs. Sunil V. Joshi and Shalmali Joshi through their Center in Nagpur, India. Contact:

Vinayak Panchakarma Chikitsalaya
Y.M.C.A. Complex Situbuldi
Nagpur (Maharastra State), INDIA 440012
Tel: 011-91-712 538983
Fax: 011-91-712-552409

For Ayurvedic Lifestyle Counseling, Drs. Sunil V. Joshi and Shalmali Joshi can be contacted through their Center in the United States:

Vinayak Ayurveda Center
2509 Virginia NE, Suite D
Albuquerque, NM 87110
Tel: 505-296-6522
Fax: 505-298-2932
Internet: www.ayur.com

CENTERS AND PROGRAMS ON AYURVEDA:

The Chopra Center for Well Being
7590 Fay Avenue, Suite 403
LaJolla, CA 92037
1-619-551-7788
1-619-551-7811 (Fax)

American Institute of Vedic Studies
P.O. Box 8357
Santa FE, NM 87504-8357
1-505-983-9385
1-505-982-5807 (Fax)

The Ayurvedic Institute and Wellness Center
11311 Menaul, NE
Albuquerque, NM 87112
1-505-291-9698
1-505-294-7572 (Fax)

Maharishi Ayurved at the Raj
1734 Jasmine Avenue
Fairfield, IA 52556
1-800-248-9050
1-515-472-2496 (Fax)

Institute for Wholistic Education
33719 116th Street, Box AP
Twin Lakes,WI 53181
1-414-877-9396

AYURVEDIC HERBS AND PRODUCTS

Vinayak Panchakarma Chikitsalaya
Y. M. C. A. Complex, Situbuldi
Nagpur (Maharastra State) India 440012
0011-91-712-538983
0011-91-712-552409 (Fax)
Retail/Wholesale

Vinayak Ayurveda Center
2509 Virginia NE, Suite D
Albuquerque, NM 87110
1-505-296-6522
1-505-298-2932 (Fax)

Siddhi Ayurvedic Beauty Products
c/o Vinayak Ayurveda Center
2509 Virginia NE, Suite D
Albuquerque, NM 87110
1-505-296-6522
1-505-298-2932 (Fax)

Internatural
33719 116th Street, Box AP
Twin Lakes, WI 53181
1-800-643-4221
Retail Mail Order

Lotus Brands, Inc.
P.O. Box 325-AP
Twin Lakes, WI 53181
1-414-889-8561
1-414-889-8591 (Fax)

Lotus Light Natural Body Care
P.O. Box 1008, Lotus Drive, Dept. AP
Silver Lake, WI 53170
1-414-889-8501 or 1-800-548-3824
1-414-889-8591 (Fax)

INDEX

AYURVEDA AND THE MIND
The Healing of Consciousness

DR. DAVID FRAWLEY

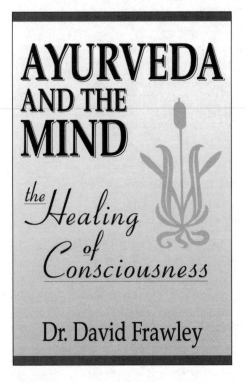

"*Ayurveda and the Mind* addresses, with both sensitivity and lucidity, how to create wholeness in Body, Mind and Spirit. This book opens the door to a new energetic psychology that provides practical tools to integrate the many layers of life. Dr. Frawley has added another important volume to his many insightful books on Ayurveda and Vedic sciences."

DEEPAK CHOPRA M.D.
AUTHOR, *Ageless Body, Timeless Mind*

PUBLISHED BY LOTUS PRESS
To order your copy, send $19.95 plus $3.00 postage and handling
($1.50 each add'l copy) to:
> Lotus Press
> P.O.Box 325AP
> Twin Lakes, WI 53181
> Request our complete book and sidelines catalog.
> Wholesale inquiries welcome.